THE BEST OF THE REST OF BRUTALLY HUGE
THE BRUTAL YEARS

By BILL DAVIS

The Best of the Rest of Brutally Huge-The Brutal Years

Table of Contents

Foreword	Pg.2
Somewhere on the other Side of Huge	Pg.3
When Huge is Not Enough	Pg.79
30 inch Thighs and 20 inch Cows	Pg.91
Yard Wide Shoulders and 22 Inch Arms	Pg.107
How to Build a 55 inch Chest	Pg.124
Brutal Back	Pg.133
Brutal Deltoids	Pg.142
Heavily Armed	Pg.154
18 inch forearms	Pg.164
Brutal Abs	Pg.173
Measurement Chart	Pg.183

Disclaimer: Before starting any exercise routine or nutritional advice in this book. Please consult your physician.

All material in this book is copyright protected 1989. Unauthorized duplication or selling of this book in any form will be prosecuted to the fullest extent of the law.

© Bill Davis 2016

FOREWORD

I want to thank you for purchasing this fine book. What I have done is combine about nine books and booklets into one compilation book. I have done this not only as a cost savings for you the reader, but also to get out there this excellent information, which will now be readily available in one book, versus having to buy each one separately. Each book will have some overlap, which needless to say would be consistent with the Brutally Huge methodology, but will also offer brutal pearls of wisdom not found in other books, as well as different perspectives on certain bodybuilding issues. We will constantly pound home the central theme of under training, increasing rest times, intensity, and poundage's. I am not promising you a Mr. Olympia victory, only one out of 7 billion humans gets that far. I firmly believe that depending on your height, genetics, desire, and commitment to brutally intense training; that 18-21 inch arms are obtainable for most people. Yes, by adhering to the proprietary and unique information and principles found in this book, you can get larger than you ever thought possible. With the information contained in the following pages, you can be healthy and Brutally Huge for life. Best wishes and may you be Brutally Huge for life.

SOMEWHERE ON THE OTHER SIDE OF HUGE

Table Of Contents

Personal Story	Pg.4
Reason For The Course	Pg.6
Overtraining	Pg.8
Undertraining	Pg.14
Steroids	Pg.17
Genetics	Pg.22
Mental Attitude	Pg.25
Intensity and Your Nerves	Pg.28
Forced Reps	Pg.30
How Worshipping Numbers Stunts Growth	Pg.32
Setting Goals	Pg.36
Stress	Pg.38
Arm Specialization	Pg.40
Description of Exercises	Pg.46
Routines: Beginner, Intermediate, and Advanced	Pg.62

PERSONAL STORY

My name is Bill, and I am the creator of How To Get Brutally Huge, and its' successor: Somewhere On The Other Side Of Huge. I have been bodybuilding for 9 years. I have trained many bodybuilders. Many people have bought the course How To Get Brutally Huge and have done just that, gotten Brutally Huge!

When I started lifting weights, I weighed 140 lbs. and had 11" arms. After taking a mandatory physical education class in junior high school; my arms went from 11 - 13" just from a year of climbing ropes, pushups, and doing a few calisthenics. Soon after, I saw the movie Pumping Iron, I realized that I had to someday look like all those bodybuilders with 20" plus arms.

I have learned a lot in my 9 years of lifting, and still have more to learn. I won't tell you to do twenty sets per body part, or take dangerous drugs, and expect you to believe that such ignorant practices will solve your lack of growth problems. The only people who can grow off 20 sets per body part are the genetically gifted, and those who use mega doses of anabolic steroids. I have undertrained from the beginning, and intuitively knew that my brand of training was sound and made provisions for the delicate recuperative powers of the body. I believe that my courses are successful for the majority of people. Tell me, how can you not grow from under training and overeating? Having this course in your hands, you have no excuse not to get huge. Read and reread the course until you thoroughly understand all of the principles contained in it.

REASON FOR THE COURSE

There is a reason for Somewhere On The Other Side OF Huge. Being a businessman I am interested in making a profit. I am even more interested in getting huge. Furthermore, I am disgusted by the ignorance that prevails in the world of bodybuilding. 99% of you are in the dark, and you don't even know why. It is so easy to grow; if only you knew what I know. I am going to show you how easy it is to grow. Sure the pain you must endure is great, and the workouts are torturous, but the principles that allow for growth are so simple that even a 5 year old could understand them.

I really want to see all of you get as huge as possible, and I want to see you do it with your health intact, and with minimal investment in time and money. My courses are based on scientific principles; more to the point; they are based on the inability of the human body to respond and grow from gross amounts of exercise. Gross amounts of exercise are those such as the marathon workouts practiced by 99% of bodybuilders. The Brutally Huge courses are based on recuperation and under training. Get it straight now; as long as you continue to over train you will never get huge, period! Your average bodybuilding routine is based on ignorance not scientific fact. A bodybuilder achieves a 17" arm, continues overtraining, doesn't grow for a year, so he reasons that he has hit his genetic potential, and now must use drugs if he desires further growth. How incorrect and illogical that thinking is! Congratulations on buying this course; now you have a chance to get huge, and stay healthy doing so.

OVERTRAINING

The whole basis of the brutally huge system is the avoidance of overtraining, or more specifically under training is what you want to do. When you over train you will never grow. You may even lose size and strength when you over train. A lot of people who go on drugs, and then add even more sets destroy a certain amount of "real tissue"; even though their measurements are going up due to the water retention from the steroids. When they go off the steroids they wonder why they are smaller than when they started the drugs. Assuming you are eating enough, and going to failure; then the only reason you are not growing is because of overtraining. As long as you over train you will never grow, and you will blame it on you having reached your genetic potential, and then you will have the excuse you need to use drugs, which is something you should not ever want to do! Zero growth can be attributed to overtraining 99% of the time.

I am not the originator of this type of exercise physiology, but after a workout your body goes through 3 steps: First, the body regains lost energy spent on doing the workout. Secondly, your body repairs the damage you did to it from the workout. It is during the second phase that your body will build itself back to the same measurement it was on the day of the workout. Have you ever noticed that on the day after the workout that you feel smaller then on the day of the workout? Thirdly, if you allow enough time to elapse, growth will occur. Think about this: if you are losing size and strength; then you probably aren't even reaching stage 2 because if you were you'd always at least be the same size. However you are losing it; then you aren't completing the second stage of recuperation. If for example, your arms are 18", but they aren't shrinking or growing, but are always 18"; then you are completing stage 2, but aren't completing or even starting stage 3. This happens because you aren't allowing enough time between workouts. When you have that magical, expansive feeling; then you know you are completing phase 3. If you always feel thick and tight; then there is obviously no problem with your recuperation; however, you might not be performing each set hard enough, or you might not be consuming enough calories. A good example: let's say you are on a training routine, and your bodyweight is going up, and your legs are growing, but your arms aren't. Then obviously you just aren't training your arms hard enough, or you could be overtraining them. Since your weight is going up; then it can't be your diet that is the problem. Let me give you another example: if your arms are 20"; then if you train them on Monday, on Tuesday they might be a little sore. On Wednesday or even Thursday they will be feeling kind of okay. By Friday they will feel tight and thick, and when you flex a tricep, or bicep it will sort of jam and cramp up. You will feel when it is growing. On Friday or Saturday they will be ready to work again.

Your body completes its growth and repair process at its own rate. Your body doesn't care about your workout program or if you're suppose to work out again on Friday, when your body is still sore. The recovery process isn't mediated or dictated by your workout calendar of events. It does what it has to, and that could take 3,4, or even 6 days , so if you want to grow you will have to build your routines around the body's recuperative powers, not when some man made routine says that your body will recover in 2 days just because you're supposed to work legs on Monday and Thursday for example. If you work them on Monday and they aren't fully recuperated on Thursday, and you go ahead and work them anyway; then you just interrupted the growth process, and congratulations, you won't grow. Your body parts will grow when they are darn good and ready to, not because you want to work them out again. Have I made this point thoroughly clear? The only thing you can do to speed up the process is to rest a lot, be of peace of mind and body, and consume a lot of calories.

The more sets you do the more you will over train. What do you think you are made of, some unlimited reserve of energy? The more you over train, the longer it will take to recuperate. I suppose you could grow from 20 set workouts if you were to rest 6 to 12 days before working that body part again? You can't grow from overtraining. When will you learn this? If everybody in the world knew what I do; then they'd all have 20" arms. I feel that all the thousands of wasted dollars and hours that I will save you is worth the price of this course. I believe in this material that strongly.

At the intermediate to advanced stage, if you are sore to the touch, then you over trained. You should only be stiff after workouts, not raw or sore to the touch. The only time you should be sore is after a layoff, or when you have been shocked by a new routine, or exercise. Look to overtraining for almost all your growth problems. If you are not losing weight; then you must be eating enough to at least maintain it. So diet isn't the culprit. If you are going to failure on the last set of an exercise; then you are obviously training hard enough. Overtraining is usually the culprit when you eliminate all the other variables.

If you bought this course thinking that I was going to insult your intelligence by telling you that simply doing 20 sets more than you are doing now will solve all your lack of growth problems; then you are wrong. This chapter that you have just read is probably the most important one in the whole course. I have seen people who nutritionally have done everything wrong, they walk in the gym and perform a few sets of bench presses, and their pecs and triceps just get huge. On the other side of the room is some little guy doing all his flyes, cable crossovers, pec decs, bench presses, and who knows what else in the mistaken belief that he must work the muscles from all angles to get a good workout. Yeah, he got a good workout alright. As a matter of fact, it was good for only one thing......NO GROWTH! Avoidance of overtraining will do more for you than drugs, diet, intensity methods, or anything else you can think of for that matter.

I'll admit that psychologically it feels like you had a better workout when you do more exercises, but believe me you won't grow. It doesn't feel good to do only 5 sets for your pecs; then go home. That is what Arnold meant by staying hungry. If you leave the gym saying wow, I feel like I did enough; then you can bet that your last protein pill that you over trained. If, however, you leave the gym with the feeling of not having done as much as you wanted to do; then you will have a better chance of growing. The choice is yours. Do you want to have good workouts, and stay puny, or do you want to train the right way, and get huge? Think about it.

UNDERTRAINING

I am going to stress this subject throughout this course. Maybe one of you will have enough faith, and want to grow bad enough that you will at least give these methods a try. Of course there are always the "know it alls", despite the fact that their arms are still only 15, 16, or maybe 17" around. Those of you who have bought this course have already shown that your minds are at least open enough to read this through; despite the fact that I probably won't tell you things that you want to hear. Once you have mastered the art and science of under training, there is no limit to how big you can get. Through under training, you will experience non-stop growth. I'm not promising you miracles, just nonstop growth.

In a few words here are the 5 steps that will get you huge:

1) UNDERTRAINING
2) DESIRE
3) PROGRESSIVE OVERLOAD
4) PROPER NUTRITIONAL HABITS
5) BELIEVING IN YOURSELF

Under training is the key. If you are doing 8 to 12 sets for your biceps now, and they aren't growing; then why don't you add 10 more sets of bicep training to your current routine? A month later when they still haven't grown; then add 10 more sets to that routine. Next month when you still haven't grown, then add 10 more sets to your bicep routine. Why don't you even quit your job, dump your friends, quit school, and start training 3 times a day like some of the champs do? Oh, that'll get you huge real quick......maybe in a thousand years. When your arms have shrunk an inch, and your joints hurt, and you hate your training; then maybe you'll smarten up and realize that large amounts of sets aren't the answer (at least for the natural trainer), or maybe you'll quit all together? There's a better way found in this book.

I am warning you, that later on in this course when I detail body part training and say do only 4 sets for a certain muscle; then I mean do only 4 sets. If you add even one more set than is recommended; then don't come crying to me because you haven't grown at all. 99% of bodybuilders are so set in their ways they can't learn anything new. Most bodybuilders I've met, are so ignorant that they are afraid of losing a 1/4 of an inch if they try something different, or don't "do enough sets", which almost certainly guarantees that you have over trained.

I didn't arbitrarily pick these numbers for my health. If you want to grow then listen to me and please do what I say to do. You've spent all this money, so don't waste it by not adhering to these principles. I promise you that you will get huge if you under train and do what I suggest. It is all up to you. You can keep doing the champs overtraining routines and stay tiny, or you can train my way, and grow larger than you may have thought possible. With my scientific system of under training and allowing recuperation to occur, you now have a chance to get an 18", 20", or even a 23" arm. With the "champ's" ignorant drug based routines, you didn't ever have a chance. Remember you can keep doing 10, 20, or even 30 sets per body part and never grow, and waste another 5 years of your life, or you can start all over and learn to train correctly and get Brutally Huge.

STEROIDS

I hate to even write about this subject, but everyone wants to know about them. However don't expect me to tell you what you want to hear. Steroids are potentially dangerous drugs that can cause serious health problems and even **DEATH!**

In my opinion the use of anabolic substances by otherwise healthy individuals is morally wrong. There are people all over the world, who are sickly, crippled, or diseased, and they would do anything to look like you or be in your shoes rather than dying, and you need to use drugs for the purpose of putting on another plastic inch on your arms?

First of all it is my opinion that probably 100% of the Olympians use mega doses of drugs. If they didn't, they would look more like you and I. Let's face it.....do you ever think that you'll look that way some day from the way you are progressing now? I'm not trying to plant a negative thought in your head, but if you go the natural route it make take 10, 15, or even 20 years. I have been lifting for 9 years; my arms have gone from 12 to 22 ", and they are still growing; furthermore, I am nowhere near where I want to be. That may take 9 more years, but I will be healthy, alive, and have 24" arms, and I will keep them until the day I die in a 100 years because I won't be diseased from steroid abuse, or have tumors all over my liver! Right now you are young, and all you can think about is fame and winning some Mr. Podunk trophy. Did you ever stop to think that in 15 years the last thing you will care about is some dumb trophy?

I hate to say this, but drugs do work, just look at the Olympians. Anyone who says they don't, are misinformed, and anyone who believes they don't is ignorant of the facts. However, drugs don't cause miracles. An example in point: everyone says that the Olympians all took lots of drugs, and that drugs made them what they are. Well since we all know there are millions of little bodybuilders with 16" arms taking drugs: then where are all the millions of Olympians? Drugs can turn a 19" smooth arm into a 19" to 20" ripped arm, but they probably won't add 6 inches to your 14 inch arm. And if you do take enough drugs to add that much size, you may pay a terrible price with your health someday.

Drugs can only do so much. Don't forget about genetics, persistence, under training, desire, and other intangible qualities. The Olympians would be big even without the drugs they use. They just wouldn't have such mind boggling cuts and definition. Their awesome cuts that you admire so much are like a vapor; they will disappear when they discontinue the drug therapy. Remember you must have a certain amount of natural talent first.

If you are going to be bull-headed and stupid enough to use drugs regardless; then they should only be used for maintaining mass while cutting up, not for building up large amounts of mass. Secondly, the larger you get naturally; the better they work. The longer you have trained, and the bigger you are the more muscle receptor sites you have developed. This means more hormone molecules, and consequently more protein molecules can bind to the muscle causing more growth. Steroids will work a lot better for a person who has trained naturally for 10 years, and has a 20" arm; than for someone who has trained for 4 years, and only has a 16 or 17" arm.

When you take drugs you are admitting defeat. You are admitting that you are a wimple. You are saying: "oh, I can't do it anymore on my own; I am a wimp and need drugs to help me". I can't take the hard workouts, or the pain. All that negative "I can't" crap makes me sick. All the little men who use drugs make me sick. If the use of drugs is so decent and acceptable; then why don't all these little bodybuilders go around bragging about their drug use? Have you ever noticed how they all lie, and say they've never used them? Give me a break. Almost anyone can get 18, 19, or even 20" arms. It's not genetics that prevents such size, but the ignorance, and inefficiency of most people's current training practices. If you've got any integrity, then you will try like heck to train without them! If you want the "easy" way out; then go ahead, and use them, but don't say I didn't warn you.

I'm sure some of you are saying: "well, I don't see anything happening to the champs". Well have you ever noticed that a lot of champs come and go and you never hear from them again? If blood was coming out of your penis from failing kidneys would you brag about it to your friends? If you are thinking that it can't happen to you; then I feel sorry for you. I won't lie; I hoped I have opened some of your eyes, and scared you off from a life of misery stemming from the ignorant use of drugs. Most doctors don't know that much about these drugs. What makes you so knowledgeable? Because you've stuck a few needles in your behind, or the biggest klutz in your gym says: yeah I took D-bol for 2 years, and nothing has happened yet. I've put all of this in this book because I care about your health; don't you? Lastly, I'm sorry, but having not used any drugs in my life, I can't give you any accurate advice on how to take them. My attitude is, just don't take steroids, period! Instead, let's just see how HUGE we can get you without them.

GENETICS

In my opinion genetics can make you or break you. It is also harped on too much, and overused as an excuse by the "little men" to use steroids, which they want to use anyway, but these people need an excuse to make them feel justified about their drug use. I guess reaching a plateau because of overtraining is a good excuse.

I've seen people with excellent genetics who go nowhere. I've seen people who appear to have poor genetics, but with proper nutrition, attitude, and persistence who overtook the seemingly genetically superior people. Larry Scott an Olympian was very skinny; however, he eventually built an arm measuring 20.5 inches in circumference. The lesson here is: you can't judge a book by its cover. Just because you might be skinny doesn't mean that you have poor genetics. The bigger you get; the more things usually seem to iron themselves out. If you're skinny but gain weight and size fast, do you really have poor genetics? No, of course you don't. A person with a large bone frame can hold more mass than a smaller boned person. There is a way to tell what size bone structure you have. It will give you a rough idea. If your wrists are over 8 inches; your bones are large. If your wrists are 6.5- 7.5 they are medium sized. A wrist measuring less than 6.5 inches is a small structure. However, that doesn't mean you won't ever get a 20" arm. Please note though that my wrists have gone from 7.5 to 8.5 inches in the last 9 years from all the weightlifting, and drinking a gallon of milk a day; both of which cause your bones to grow much larger. The tendons and bones do get thicker.

Genetics control hair color and eye color, it controls height, foot size, skin color, and bone structure. It even controls muscle shape. However, for your purposes, it does not control size. If you have a short bicep you'll never make it longer, but you can make the lower portion incredibly thick. Can you see the difference?

Genetics can control your growth rate to a degree. My arms have grown at the rate of 1/4" for 3 to 5 months in a row. Furthermore, this has happened many times in the last 8 years. However, it was always 1/4 " a month. Some people can add a 1/2", or 3/8" per month. Everyone is different.

No one has yet reached their potential. Scientists have proven that the genetic limit for any muscle is that it can't grow thicker than it is long. Another words, if your bicep is 9" long with your arm extended; then it can never exceed 9" in width when contracted. That is the limit. An arm with that kind of mass would easily be 30" around, so selling yourself short and training for a 24" arm, or a smaller 21" arm shouldn't be any great deal. Taking all of this into consideration it would be stupid to think that just because your arm has been stuck at 18" for a year (due to overtraining most likely) that you have reached your genetic potential. Please give me a break. The day you ever reach your potential you will be the biggest muscular freak on the face of the Earth. If you under train, overeat, and get proper rest, and recuperation; then you can't stop growth. It will happen at incredible speed. Forget genetics! Learn the art of under training.

MENTAL ATTITUDE

Mental attitude is so important when it comes to getting Brutally Huge. Believing in yourself and believing that you can get huge in the first place is probably the most important aspect of getting huge. Having an open mind is part of what is takes to get huge. One must be open to new ways of thinking and training, and to go against the common thinking of the herd mentality. How can you learn anything when you think you know it all? I get really irritated when I run into some little gym guy who has a 15" arm, and thinks that he knows it all when it comes to bodybuilding. These little fellows think that they know it all, and will even dare to challenge my knowledge in the gym. For example, there I am right in front of him with my arms at least 6 to 8" bigger than his; he then asks me what it takes to grow so large, and after I tell him, he then argues with me saying that it can't possibly work. Then why did he ask me in the first place. As a general rule of thumb; I don't help people anymore in person unless I know they are sincere and are going to try what I tell them to do. You must have an open mind if you want to get really huge. Sometimes you will hear things you won't like, or you might have to do things that you won't necessarily like to do. Sometimes it takes faith and courage to step outside of your comfort zone and try something new, especially like what'll you'll read in these books, which have nothing in common with the conventionally accepted bodybuilding "wisdom". I don't even know it all. I am still in the process of learning new information.

If you want to get big then you have to think big. As one Olympian I've met said: "think big, or don't think at all". You must live eat, and breathe the thought of getting huge, 24 hours a day. If you have an 18" arm, but want a 19" arm; then set your sights on 20", not on 19". Otherwise you might never get there. It's like the old saying, if you want to reach the moon, shoot for the stars. I want you to get huge, but first you must relearn what you thought about proper training and reprogram your mind. You have to want to get big, or otherwise you won't. Your subconscience can and will hold you back. Being huge can be difficult. Everyone is going to treat you differently. Some people will like you, some will fear you, some will be intimidated by you, some won't like how you are built, and some will like you just as you are. Mentally speaking, you can't let what other people think of you, hold you back. There were times where other's opinion of what I was doing affected me in a negative way. Sometimes, it actually slowed down my growth process. Now I live for the day when my arms will stretch the tape to 24 inches, and I don't care what other people think. Please be cautious of envious small minded people who will put you down and try to hold you back in life because of their own insecurities. Surround yourself by like minded positive people who won't try to keep you down. Remember, when you succeed, you are a constant reminder of negative little minded people's own failures and inadequacies. Sometimes it helps to use your imagination in colorful ways. You have to imagine yourself being so huge that it looks like you are in pain when you are walking around. They will have to wheel you out on the stage. If you don't believe that you can get huge then you never will. Your mind can stunt all growth if it is negatively programmed. Indeed, your own mind can be your worst enemy. I can guarantee that probably at least 95% of you are genetically capable of building at least an 18, or 19" arm, but you've got to believe it and believe in yourself.

INTENSITY

I would like to briefly touch upon the subject of intensity. Too much of a good thing can ruin your training efforts. Too much intensity can even halt or reverse growth so that you shrink. You see, it is not only your muscles that need a long rest after a brutal workout. Your nerves need a lot of rest too. How many of you have done heavy squats on a Monday, and then on the next leg workout, you are dreading doing them? You say: "I don't feel like squatting". Your nerves and endocrine systems are still shot from that last workout. Your adrenals and your nerves can get fried real easily from doing too much intensity, too often. It is like the guy who does forced reps on every set and is raw the next day. I routinely see lifters doing 6 or 7 forced reps on the bench press with a weight they were only able to do once or twice. I tried supersets for my biceps once for about 2 weeks, and for those two weeks they were growing like crazy; then around the third week I noticed that the same routine was not producing any results. I noticed that my arms were feeling puny; sure enough they softened up and lost about 1\8 to 1\4 of an inch. I was too stubborn or inflexible to quit and go back to straight sets for a period of time and take it easy on myself for a while. Now I know better. Intensity methods should be used very sparingly. You should always go to positive failure on the heaviest and last set of an exercise. You may do 1 cheat rep or 1 forced rep at the end of such a set, but no more otherwise you run the risk of overtraining. The more intensity that you employ in your own training; the more you must decrease the overall number of sets that you can do. In other words, intensity and workout volume are inversely related. Furthermore, as intensity increases, you must also rest more days in between such harshly demanding workouts. To sum it up, if you are not growing, maybe you are training too intensely too much of the time, and are perhaps burned out. Think about it!

FORCED REPS

Let's talk about the issue of forcing growth to occur. Everyone acts like getting muscles to grow is such a difficult task. Growth is only difficult because most of you keep adding more sets, more intensity methods, and other techniques that fry your nerves, and prevent you from growing. Have you ever noticed that even though your biceps may feel fine 2 to 3 days after a workout that you still feel lethargic and burned out? That is because your nerves and the systems that allow growth to occur are still doing their work, but you won't let them finish if you keep training to often.

Muscles are like gasoline. It doesn't take a massive explosion to set off a tank of gasoline; just one little spark will do that. Growth is the same way. A muscle just needs a little bit of stimulation, and if they are allowed to rest, they will grow. More often than not muscle growth must be coaxed not forced. When you can only bench 205lbs for 2 reps, but you force out 4,5,6, or even 7 more reps; then not only are you exposing yourself to overtraining, exposing your joints to trauma, but you are also overtaxing the systems that allow for growth to occur. It doesn't take mega loads of intense effort to cause a muscle to grow; all it takes is making the muscle do a little more than it is normally accustomed to doing. You should never do more than one or two forced reps on a particular exercise, and then; you should only do it on the last and heaviest set. If you insist on doing more than that you will only over train, you will not grow.

WHY WORSHIPPING NUMBERS STUNTS GROWTH

You will find that a lot of this course deals with the intangible, things that aren't concrete, things you can't see, feel, or understand. A lot of this course deals with the mind. Chances are that many of you; when you first saw the advertisement for Somewhere on the Other Side of Huge; thought that there was going to be a 1oo plus pages of all kinds of secret exercises. Well I hate to inform you of this, but there are no secret exercises, well sometimes you can invent something weird that no one else does. The secret must come from within. It is based on how your mind operates. I would go so far as to say, that the mind is the most important thing when it comes to growth on a large scale. The mind is probably even more important than diet or exercise. Your exercise can be hard, your diet sufficient in nutrients, but if your mind isn't with it you just won't extract maximum benefit.

Let's talk about measurements and worshipping numbers. When the mind is with it, you can grow by leaps and bounds, but when it is against you, nothing you do can make you grow. Setting goals such as arm measurements are very important when it comes to growing. Goals give you a reason to exist, if you will.

Goals give you something to strive for; otherwise you would soon stagnate, and spin your wheels in the sands of bodybuilding non-progress. Psychologically though, there is a problem with worshipping numbers, or measurements. You see, when you worship a number you are (in a way you can't realize) putting yourself below the number and placing an invisible barrier upon yourself. You are putting the number up on a pedestal, and almost worshipping it. When you say, or think things like: "oh, I'll never get a 20" arm then chances are you won't. You have already defeated yourself before you have given it a chance. When will you realize that 20" is a number just like 14, 16, 19, 19.75, or even 23 inches? No one has ever reached their genetic potential; so how dare anyone try to tell you that a 20" arm is the genetic limit for any member of the human race. When you place limits of the negative kind like this on yourself, it is hard to reach the 20" arm let alone surpass it. You must stop worshipping numbers right now, and tell yourself that a number is just a number. They don't mean anything.

In Karate when you take lessons in self defense they tell you to follow through. More specifically when you are performing a punch; let's say a punch to someone's face; you don't aim for his face; you aim for a point behind his head, and then punch with all the force you can develop. By the time you arm has straightened out the poor guy is laying flat on his back.

The same thing must be done when you are trying to break through goals and measurements. If you want a 20" arm, but right now you have a 19" arm; then don't think of the number 20". That is placing a mental, and therefore a physical limit on yourself. If you have a 19" arm, and you want a 20" arm; then set your goals on 20.5" or maybe 21". You see you won't get a 21" arm when you do this, but subconsciously thinking of 21" will make you think that 20" is no big deal, and that maybe somehow you have all ready done it. Keep thinking 21", 21", 21", 21", 21". The more you think of the number 21" the less you will worry about the small number 20". It's using a kind of mental trickery on yourself.

A 20" arm is only a big deal to those who don't have one. How many of you out there reading this course have 17" arms? It's no big deal is it? Do you remember though a while back when you only had a 15" arm and how you thought 17" was the world? Well as hard as this may be for you to comprehend; a 20" arm means nothing to me. You see, they have been over

20" for so long now that I have forgotten what it is like to be that small. Actually I'm just kidding a 20" arm is not small, but it is not big either, and furthermore it is not your genetic limit. Size is relative. It depends on who is doing the talking. You see, a 16" arm is small to someone who has a 18" arm, but it is huge to someone who has a 14" arm. So, it really depends on how you look at it. I know you don't believe me now, but I hope someday that you do get a 20" arm, and then have it for a year, which will give you enough time to acclimate yourself to your new size, and make you realize that yes, Bill Davis was right about a 20" arm being no big deal. So, from now on set numerical goals, but don't place them so far above yourself that you can't believe in it yourself, or ever achieve them. Never again look at a mere number as some kind of idol, something that is unattainable.

SETTING GOALS

Setting goals is very important in the game of muscle growth. Setting goals helps you to get where you want to be a lot faster. If you didn't have goals you would be lost. Without goals you will have no direction. How can you begin a course of action with no goals to shoot for? Goals give you a reason to live as well as to train. In the process of setting a goal you automatically must take a course of action that will initiate the self fulfilling prophecy that will start a chain reaction of complex events that will eventually get you there.

Start off with small, reasonable, easy to obtain goals. Your arm is only 15"; I know that you want a 21" arm, but first you must set a goal to conquer the 16" arm. Once you have reached that goal; then you may shoot for the 17" arm. The more goals you set and conquer the more confidence that you will build. As you get bigger, and bigger; you will be more easily able to envision a 21" arm than when you had a 15" arm. Like the old Chinese proverb says: the longest journey begins with the first step. Be patient and set goals that you yourself will believe. If you can't believe in your own goals; then you will never get there, period! Also be sure to take into account genetic factors that you can't control; for instance, if you are only 5 feet tall then a 18" arm might be more reasonable to obtain than a 22" arm. However if you are 6 feet tall then you might be able to obtain a 24" arm if you under train and go about it the right way. If you have two bodybuilders, and they are both 6 feet tall, but one has thick bones while the other has frail bones; it stands to reason that the heavier boned person will probably be able to hold more skeletal mass than the smaller boned individual. Summing it up, when setting your goals take all factors into consideration.

STRESS

There are two kinds of stress: positive and negative. A positive stress might be proper bodybuilding which will cause you to grow. A negative stress is anything that keeps you from growing. You must avoid overtraining, alcohol, drugs, smoking, lack of sleep, personal problems, or whatever else is wrong in your life. When you go to the gym you must leave your problems at home. Besides, they are not going to go away in 1 or 2 hours anyway. Your problems will be there waiting for you when you are done with the workout. So, forget them for a couple of hours.

Stress in its' most severe form can kill you. In its' milder form stress can cause all kinds of real and imaginary problems, and ailments. Stress can cause ulcers, headaches, and make you so run done that you are prone to all kinds of illnesses. It can make you susceptible to infections, nervous breakdowns, and so much more. None of this is conducive to a happy, healthy life, or growth. Laughter is the best medicine. You should try to laugh hard every day. Even the bible says in one part (proverbs) that laughter is like good medicine. Stress can make you susceptible to overtraining, injuries, cessation, and even reversal of gains in size and strength. Stress can also be in the form of too many forced reps, sets, and other intensity methods. To grow at an optimum pace; then you should live by this rule: Anything that causes negative stress in your life, try to eliminate it!

ARM SPECIALIZATION

If you really want your arms to get big; then you'll love this routine. I have a 55" chest, and 21" arms. My chest is so large though; that sometimes it looks too big next to my arms. I believe that if my chest never grew again; 2 more inches on my arms would not hurt my proportions. I want arms that are slightly too big. Some of the most famous Olympians of all time had arms that were too big. Arms are number one to me. I don't want the bottom heavy look, the barrel chest look, or the slope-shouldered traps that are too big look. I want to have outrageously huge arms. At this time in my life I am following this routine:

Workout A-Legs\back\biceps\forearms
Workout B-Calves\Abs\Chest\Shoulders\ Triceps

The days of the week that I was doing this workout were:

Day	Mon	Tue	Wed	Thur	Fri	Sat	Sun	Mon	Tue	Wed
Workout	A	Rest	B	Rest	Rest	A	Rest	B	Rest	rest

There are a couple of things that you must understand though.

1) Heavy leg work stimulates your whole body to grow.

2) As your bodyweight goes up, your arms seem to grow better.

So we don't want to stop leg work, and we want to gain weight. If you are having difficulty growing your arms, then for starters, arms must be worked first and hardest. You should also realize that all those chest and back exercises are pushing your arms further and further into the overtraining zone. Chest and back work must be cut down to a bare minimum, but not stopped; as heavy chest and back work do stimulate the arms.

However since our arms are the most important here, our thinking must change. You must ask yourselves what exercises will pack on arm mass, but at least maintain the torso muscles (chest and back)? Dips, close grip benches, underhand chin-ups, and underhand pull downs are but a few. Don't be surprised if your chest and back grow better than ever from all the under training.

Here is how the system is now broke down to prioritize your arms:

Day 1

Thighs-4 sets

Hamstrings-2 sets

Day 2

Abs-2 sets

Chest-1 to 2 sets

Calves-2 to 3 sets   Triceps-1 to 2 sets

Traps-2 sets   Back-1 to 2 sets

Delts-2 sets   Forearms-2 sets

Exact example exercises could be:

<u>Day 1</u>   <u>Day 2</u>

Squats-4 sets   Weighted sit ups-2 sets
Leg curls-2 sets   close grip benches-1 to 2 sets
Calf raises-2-3 sets   lying tricep extensions-2 sets
Shrugs-2 sets   underhand chins-1 to 2 sets
Lateral raises-2 sets preacher curls-1 to 2 sets
Bent laterals-2 sets   wrist curls-1 to 2 sets
                       reverse wrist curls-1 to 2 sets

1) The workouts, if you notice, either focus on arms, or legs; keeping the blood in the vicinity.

2) If you notice that the arm work provides plenty of indirect stimulation for the torso muscles; providing you train the arms heavy as you can. Let me elucidate the theme. You can do a maximum of 4 sets of direct and indirect work combined for triceps and biceps. For example, you could do 2 sets of curls, and 1 set of underhand pull downs to failure. Trust me your lats will get pumped and will at least be maintained in size. For triceps, you could do 2 sets of Tricep press downs, the first set being a

warm up of 15-20 reps with the second set going to failure, followed by a set of dips to failure. Your pecs will pump from this and probably be maintained. Remember, this type of training is not to grow pecs and lats, but to specialize on arms, for people who are growing everywhere else just fine, but whose arms are lagging in comparison. Or, you can do 2 sets of a direct tricep movement, followed by 2 sets of a compound movement that incorporates both pecs and triceps and you can do 2 sets of a direct bicep movement followed by 2 sets of a compound movement that works both the biceps and lats. On each of the 2 sets, the first set is the higher rep warm up set, and the second set is performed to failure.

Here would be an example "bicep" workout that would also maintain your lats:

Strict barbell curls leaning against a wall-1st set is 15 reps, the 2nd set would be the heaviest weight you can do for 4-6 reps. Perform slow deliberate reps and feel your biceps burn with this one.

Followed by:

One arm dumbbell rows-the 1st set would be 6-8 reps, followed by a 2nd set of 4 reps. No heaving the weight here. Do slow deliberate reps and hold the dumbbell against your chest a couple of seconds at the top of the movement before lowering it.

Now here would be an example "tricep" workout that would also maintain your pectorals:

Tricep press down-the 1st set would be a 15-20 rep warm up (for the elbows). The 2nd set would be a fairly heavy weight you can get 6-8 strict reps out of. Perform these strictly, slowly, and feel the pain. An added tip: When performing pressdowns, lean slightly backwards and not forward and your triceps will really pump up, and you'll eliminate the pecs from helping.

Followed by:

Close grip bench presses with elbows tucked in. The 1st set would be a warm up set of 10 reps, followed by a 2nd set with the heaviest weight you can get 4-6 reps out of (with a spotter).

Legs are done by themselves, and furthermore, there is no fear of having to pace yourself because you might be too tired for arms afterwards (as in a typical Leg/Back/Bicep split).

Arms are worked first, hardest, and by themselves. As a matter of fact, if you wish to stick to the traditional leg/back/bicep and chest shoulder/tricep regimen, then to put priority on your arms, simply do them backwards. Namely, do a bicep/back/leg workout and a tricep/shoulder/chest workout in that order. Notice how the biceps and triceps would get worked first, when you are the most fresh!

Do the routine as long as you want your arms to keep on growing. This routine is especially good if your arms are a lagging body part, or you'd just like to pack on an inch real quick. Mine grew a 1/2 inch in the first month; give it a try.

EXERCISES

THIGH EXERCISES

Squats-This exercise mainly works the belly of the thighs. Among the muscles affected are the: Vastus Lateralis, Vastus Medialis, Rectus Femoris, Sartorius, Gluteus Maximus, Spinal Erectors, Traps hamstrings, and even the ribcage is expanded. Place the bar across your traps; keep your shoulder blades crunched together, so the traps bunch up to provide a cushion for the bar; keep your feet shoulder width apart, keep your head straight forward, take in a deep breath, and slowly sink down all the way to the bottom; don't bounce! Once you hit the bottom explode upwards!

Variations:

Flat footed squats- affect mostly middle and upper thighs.

Heels on board- middle and lower thighs

Feet far apart- affects thigh belly and inner thighs

Feet together- Affects frontal and side thighs

Barbell Hack Squats- If you don't have a machine you can use a barbell. Stand in front of the bar, with the back of your calves touching the bar, and you back straight; squat down just far enough to grab the bar, and once you have explode upwards. Take in a deep breath and repeat for the required number of reps. This exercise is excellent for the lower and lower outer thighs.

Variation:

At or near the top of the movement throw your hips forward. This will hit the upper thighs. Using a board will stress the knee area more. Using no board will stress the middle and outer thigh. For best results use a shoulder width stance.

Leg Press

The Leg Press will work the upper thighs. Placing your feet far apart will stress the groin area; placing them close together will hit the outside sweep. Always do full slow repetitions no matter what type of leg press apparatus you use. When your legs go to failure you can push them even further by putting your hands on your knees and pushing with them, once your thighs have hit failure on their own.

Leg Extensions

Leg Extensions are worthless for mass. These are mostly a shaping movement. Squeeze hard at the top and lower slowly Extensions will etch detail into the vastus medialis and rectus femoris.

HAMSTRING EXERCISES

Standing leg curls-Done 1 leg at a time. Placing your legs outward will hit the inner hamstrings; your feet inward will hit the outer hamstrings.

Lying Leg Curls- Keep your hips flat on the bench. It's harder, but you'll feel the hamstrings contracting harder at the top of the movement. Hamstrings like high reps done to failure.

Stiff Leg Dead lifts- Standing erect with a bar in front of you, and your legs slightly bent; lean forward until your back is parallel to the floor. Don't go down further otherwise your back rounds out, and you could hurt it on the way up.

The hamstring raise- This is the ultimate hamstring exercise. Lay face down on the floor. Have someone hold your ankles firmly. Place your hands behind your head; at the knee, raise your whole body up , and keep it straight. Add a light bar when you can do 8 to 10 reps.

CALVES

Standing Calve Raises- On the smith machine, or bar across your shoulders, or on the standing calf machine. The knees must be locked at all parts of the movement. Training in this manner will affect the gastrocnemius. As soon as you bend your knees, the soleus takes over. Squeeze hard at the top, lower all the way down; always keeping your knees locked. Positioning your heels out works the inner calves, heels in works the outer calves. Don't bounce. Do high reps. Calves respond best to lots of reps and pain. Keep the knees locked and contract hard at the top!

<u>Seated calve raise</u>- Using a machine, or bar across your knees with a towel around it. Raise the weight as high as it will go; hold for 2 seconds, slowly lower and repeat. Don't bounce! Heels out hits the inner soleus, heels in hits the outer soleus.

<u>Toe Press</u>- on the Leg Press- This exercise hits the upper calf too! Keep your knees locked. If you feel your hamstrings pulling it's because they are too tight. Toe press the weight as far as it'll go, and slowly let it stretch back. Do partials until no movement is possible at all; after you've done full reps to failure.

<u>Tibialis Anterior</u>- (shin) - Sit on the floor, hook a floor pulley to your feet (use curling handles and slide them over your shoe), and contract your feet toward you, contract; then slowly lower, and repeat for the required number of reps.

ERECTORS

Dead lifts-Load the bar with weight. Stand behind the bar. Squat down at the thighs, and grab the bar using a reverse grip. The hand you write with should be in the overhand grip. The other hand should be in the underhand position. Looking straight ahead stand up straight and as you come near the completion of the rep draw the shoulder blades back and squeeze them together. This exercise will work your erectors, traps, inner back, and even your forearms from gripping on to the weight.

<u>Hyperextensions</u>- This exercise will blast your erectors and secondarily your hamstrings. Hook the back of your feet under the pads, and arch up to a 45 degree angle above parallel. Lower to a position of 45 degrees below parallel. Add weight whenever possible.

<u>Weighted good mornings</u>- This hits your erectors and hamstrings. Assume a standing position; place the bar on your back. Keeping your back slightly arched backward, lower your torso down to almost parallel to the floor. Keep your knees slightly bent. You should feel your hamstrings pulling to. Don't be afraid to add weight, I've used as much as 290 lbs for 3 reps.

TRAPS

<u>Barbell Shrugs</u>- Holding a bar at arm's length, shrug the bar up as high as you can, attempting to touch the ears with your shoulders. Don't roll your shoulders back as this only works the inner back. Shrug it up as high as you can. This technique is what adds height to the traps.

<u>Pulls</u>-this is really a cheating upright row. Holding a bar at arms length with a medium wide grip, squat down a few inches; then explosively squat back up, and as you do, let the momentum help you pull the weight up to your lower pecs. No farther is really necessary. Three sets are all you will need with this exercise. It also works the delts, biceps, and upper forearms to a degree.

<u>Dumbbell Shrugs</u>- Use the same techniques as the barbell shrugs but you are now using db's instead of a barbell. It is for variation sake only.

<u>Upright rows</u>- Using a barbell or cable. This is supposed to be a strict movement. With a 10 "grip, deliberately pull the weight up to your chin, and hold for a few seconds. As you do this, make sure you shrug your shoulders up at the completion of the rep.

LATISSIMUS DORSI

Barbell Rows- Standing on a block that is 6" in height, bend over at the waist without rounding your back, and keep your knees slightly bent. Keep your hands about 10" apart. While looking straight ahead pull the bar to your waist, not your chest. This is the number one exercise for thickness in the lats. 3 sets are sufficient.

1 arm dumbbell rows- Bending over at the waist, place your free hand on a bench. While looking straight ahead, and pull the dumbbell to your waist. Hold it there for a second; then slowly lower. This exercise will pack on mass onto the lower lats.

Dumbbell Pullovers-This exercise will work the part of your lats right under your armpits, and it will also work the serratus, and expand the ribcage. Lie across the bench, your shoulders touching the bench, and with the weight over your face, slowly lower it behind your head. Always take in a deep breath at the start of each rep, exhale and raise back to the starting position.

Cable lat pull downs- Sit down on a bench and hook your knees under the t-bar. Grab the overhead bar with about a 2 foot grip. No wider!

Pull it down to your chin, hold, and then let it back up slowly. 2 sets are enough.

<u>Close grip underhand pull downs</u>- Same as above, but you are now using a 6-8" underhand grip. Pull it down to your chin, squeeze the lats and biceps, and feel them burn. If you do this exercise two sets are enough.

PECS

<u>Bench Press</u>- hits the middle pecs, front delts, and the triceps. Keep your feet on the floor, and keep your butt on the bench. Take in a deep breath, and slowly lower it to the area around your nipples, pause and push it back up. Don't ever bounce or injury could result! 4 sets are good here. I'd suggest a pyramid of 15, 10, 8, 6 reps. Add weight whenever possible.

<u>Incline Press</u>- Hits the upper pecs, frontal delts, and the triceps. Lift the weight off the rack, and slowly lower it to your clavicle area, hold and explosively push it back up. As you press the weight up, it is correct to push it up and back at the same time. A close grip will hit the inner pecs and a wide grip will hit the outer, upper pecs. If you do some other exercise for your chest; then 2 to 3 sets are enough here.

Decline Press- I prefer to use a smith machine because all you have to do is push the weight straight up and down. There are no problems with having to balance it. This exercise works your lower pecs. A wide grip will hit the outer, lower pecs, and a narrow grip will hit the inner, lower pecs. A medium grip is best for overall lower pec results. At the completion of each rep, kind of shrug the bar up. In other words, "pec shrug" the weight up another inch or two.

Flyes- whether on a flat, incline, or decline bench will hit the outer pecs. Hold the dumbbells at arm's length over your face, and in wide circular arcs of movement, let the weight travel out to the sides of your face. The key here is not how low the db's go, but how far down your elbows go down. Perform these very slowly.

Pec Decs- And other similar machines work the inner pecs. The key point is the contraction. At the completion of each rep you must squeeze the handles together as hard as you can, and then hold them there for a count of 2 or 3 seconds.

Db Presses- are an alternative to using barbells as they give a much better stretch.

DELTS

The 1 arm Lateral- Grab an upright with your free hand, and hold the dumbbell in the other hand. Bend your arms slightly, and raise the dumbbell out to the side about face level. The cheat principle works well on this exercise, and the side delts really respond to heavier weights versus strict light weights. I have used 110 pounders on this exercise on the last set for a few reps. Try to resist it on the way down. Two sets is sufficient.

Lateral raises- are the same as above but now you are using two db's. Lean slightly forward, so it hits your side delts. Your palms should always be facing the floor. Lower them slowly. Only 2 sets are needed.

Standing Military Presses- Lift a barbell off a rack with a slightly wider than shoulder width grip. Press it straight overhead without leaning back at all. As the set approaches failure cheat a little by squatting down a few inches and then blast back up. This exercise works the anterior delts and you should wear your belt on this one to give support to your spine.

Seated Press behind the Neck- Sitting on a bench, hold the bar with a grip so close that your thumbs are touching the side of your delts.

The most important thing is to lean slightly forward as you press the weight up on each rep. Don't use one of those seated press benches that you can lean on. They are for wimps and because you are resting and leaning slightly back the work is shifted to your front delts. The press behind the neck is suppose to work the side, rear delts, and traps.

<u>Bent over lateral raises</u>-Bend over so that your torso is parallel to the ground. Grab 2 dumbbells. Raise them out to the sides and try to get your elbows up as high as possible. Slowly lower and repeat. This exercise works the rear delts. It even hits the inner back.

<u>Lying rear laterals</u>- are the same as above but now you are lying face down on a bench and don't have to worry about balance or your lower back. On both exercises, only 2 sets are needed.

TRICEPS

<u>Dips</u>- keep your elbows tucked in, head up, and lower all the way down slowly; come back up slowly and contract the rear triceps head. This exercise is the best rear tricep exercise there is. This will make your arms look big from the sides. Two sets is perfect.

Close Grip Benches (with the elbows out to the sides)-Lying on your bench, grab the bar with a 10-12" wide grip, keeping the elbows directly out to the sides, lower the bar to your upper pectoral region, pause, and push it back up. This is one of the most excellent side tricep exercises there is. For extra growth, try not locking out at the top. This particularly hits the lower side tricep.

Close grip benches with the elbows in- Same as above but keep your elbows tucked in to the sides of your body, and lower the bar to your lower pec region. This exercise works the lower portion of the rear triceps. Do 2 sets, do each rep deliberately, with no bouncing.

Tricep Press downs- Keeping your elbows pinned in at the sides, press the weight down in a circular arc. The only thing that should move is the forearms. For a really good pump, step back away from the machine so the cable is not going straight up and down, but back at an angle. Also, try keeping your upper body erect. Don't lean into the movement. This exercise hits the lateral triceps. Two sets is more than sufficient.

Lying extensions- While lying on a bench, hold a bar over your forehead, at arm's length with about a 8 inch grip, and slowly lower it to your forehead, pause; then press it back up. Control it all the way and purposely build up the tension in your triceps.

1 arm lying extension- Same as above but one or two dumbbells are used. If you were using two dumbbells, your palms will be facing each other. Lower them to your forehead; now instead of raising them back up, let them down like you were doing pullovers; then raise them all the way up. This exercise will hit the rear triceps. Two sets is more than enough.

IMPORTANT NOTICE- ON ALL EXTENSION MOVEMENTS WHEN THE REP IS DONE IT SHOULD BE OVER YOUR FOREHEAD, AND NOT OVER YOUR CHEST.

Seated Tricep Press- Sitting on a bench, grab a bar with a 8-10" wide grip behind the head, and with your elbows directly out to the sides; press it up. High reps to failure seem to work best on this exercise. This exercise really blasts the rear triceps as well as the lower portion. Do 2 sets, perform each rep slowly, no bouncing!

BICEPS

Barbell Curls- Grab a bar with a medium wide grip, keeping the elbows purposely tucked in at the sides and curl it up. If your elbows ever go forward then you are working the anterior delts.

A close grip hits more of the outer biceps, and a wide grip gets the inner area. Deliberately curl the weight up; never cheat until you can no longer do any strict reps. The barbell curl is excellent for power and overall mass. As you curl always keep the wrists straight. If you don't, you may feel it more in your forearms. Only do 2-3 sets of this movement.

Barbell Preacher Curls-Now you are using a bench set at a particular angle; usually a 60 degree angle is the best for a peak contraction effect. This exercise will hit the lower biceps; never let it bounce at the bottom or you could tear the bicep insertion. Do slow reps and use deliberation in initiating each rep. Do 2 sets.

Underhand Chins-Hang from a bar with a 10" grip, add weight around your waist if you can, and pull up until your chin touches the bar. Contract hard, and slowly lower. This is an excellent mass builder, and you should constantly strive to add weight whenever possible. I've done chins with 105 pound Dumbbells hanging on me, and I'm not naturally strong in this movement. A strong person could and people have done chins with 200 pounds dangling on them. Two sets is enough.

Incline Db Curls- Use a bench with a 40 degree angle, lay back and while holding two dumbbells, let your arms stretch all the way back until they are hanging straight down. You might feel this pulling in your shoulders at first, but they will eventually loosen up, just take it easy. This exercise works the upper biceps. Do slow movements and feel the pain. The more pain you generate the more they will grow. Two sets should be enough.

FOREARMS

Reverse Barbell Curls- Stand with a barbell hanging at arms length in front of your thighs, and using an overhand grip about 10" wide curl the weight. As you curl the weight up only your forearms should move. This exercise works the Brachioradialis, which is situated on the upper outer forearm. Try a kamber bar for variation.

Wrist Curls- Sit on a bench. Rest both forearms on the bench and use your thighs to keep them clamped together. Only your hands should be hanging over the bench, and they should be able to move freely up and down. Do high reps, and do them strictly, and go to failure, and when full reps are no longer possible; then do partials, and partial partials to failure. They should burn like hell. With this kind of torture, 2 sets will be more than you want to do.

Reverse wrist curls- are the opposite of the above movement. Your hands should now be facing the floor. Do high reps and go to failure. Go all the way up and all the way down, and always go as heavy as you can. Squeeze each rep at the top, 1-2 sets is good.

Standing Wrist Curls-Grab a bar behind your waist and curl the weight up and down using the fullest range of motion. This is kind of an awkward movement, but it really blasts the lower forearms.

ABS

Leg Raises Works the lower abs. Let your butt and legs hanging over a bench, knees slightly bent, raise them up and down. Don't ever bounce! Go very slow. Use tension and extra weight whenever possible. Do no more than 2 sets.

Weighted Sit ups- Works the middle abs. Hold the weight behind your head. Chin on your chest, and curl your torso inward and towards your knees. You should curls up, not sit up with your torso straight like a board. Two sets is plenty.

Weighted Crunches- Upper abs. Rules are the same as above for sit ups. But you are on a roman chair. Two sets is enough.

Note: for variation, all exercises can be done on flat, decline, or incline benches. For more extensive abdominal training techniques you might want to obtain and consult the Brutal Abs course.

ACTUAL EXERCISE ROUTINES

Thighs-Hamstrings

If you want to get big thighs you must do full squats. Full Leg Presses of any kind are excellent also. However squats are still the king of mass when it comes to building the thighs. Let us first clear up a major myth: squats, more exactly full squats will not hurt your knees as long as you don't BOUNCE, and secondly warm-up your knees. There is one exception though; if you do have bad knees; and if squats aggravate the condition... don't do them. Do slow partial squats or leg presses instead. The name of the longevity game is to avoid anything that hurts you in bodybuilding. If Mr. Olympia says: "do this kind of curl for massive biceps", but it hurts your wrists; then don't do them. Whenever possible, do full squats rather than half squats. Why is everybody so afraid to go all the way down? I'd rather do full squats with 300lbs; than do partials with 600lbs, and crunch my spinal discs. I guess doing full squats are only done by people with more fortitude, and everyone else is afraid of a little hard work. You will never get 30" thighs by doing leg extensions either. It's just like benches are better than flyes for pec mass. So if you really want to get huge thighs; then I'd suggest you do 4 sets of full squats. Here is a sample routine based on a 375-400lb full rep max:

135 x 20, 205 x 15, 275 x 10, 335 x 4-6 reps

Rules:

1) Add weight every workout if possible
2) Go all the way down extremely slow, and explode upwards.
3) Flex the thighs very hard in between sets for more pump.
4) The best thigh warm-up is a set of 50 to 100 reps on leg ext.
5) Keep your back straight and always look straight ahead
6) Never bounce! Do only slow deliberate reps!

As for hamstrings always do 2 sets of leg curls or something similar after your thigh workout. Pullovers can and should be done after leg training. This will expand the ribcage. Do 2 sets of 15 to 20 reps. Always take in the deepest breath possible preceding each rep, and hold it during the rep. So in one typical leg\back\bicep workout you have now done:

Squats 4 sets of 20, 15, 10, and 6 reps
Leg Curls 2 sets of 0 to 15 reps
Pullovers 2 sets of 15 to 20 reps

We will discuss the back and biceps later, now we will talk about calves.

CALVES

Calves are real simple to make grow. One thing you must remember is that you are on them all day long. The last thing they need is 20 sets. I've never seen anyone get huge calves from overtraining unless they were on truckloads of anabolics. What calves need are more intensity than what you would normally experience in daily life. Calves are muscles too. They need to rest a lot. You wouldn't work your biceps every day would you? I hope not! You see somewhere along the way someone said calves are stubborn, and therefore must be worked every day. Well of course they seem stubborn to respond if you do that much work for them. Standing calve raises , and toe presses on a leg press are best for mass, but don't do them both in anyone workout or you'll over train. To sum it up calves grow best from:

1)High reps to failure
2)Low number of sets

3) Ultra strict form
4) Extreme pain
5) Full reps; all the way up and down. Contract at the top and hold.

On most calf exercises your knees should be locked. As soon as you bend them even an inch the more powerful soleus comes into play. From my own empirical data I have determined that if you do more than 3 to 4 sets total for the calves they won't grow. Here is a sample routine that I presently am getting results from. I gained exactly 3\8" in May 1988 doing this routine:

Standing calves -25, 20,15 reps to failure
Seated calves-1 set with 425 lbs for 4 to 6 reps
Tibialis anterior raises-2 sets of 10, 6 reps

Forget all that stupid bouncing up and down in between sets thinking it is going to stretch your calves or make them grow, or something. You should've stretched them during the set with 400 pounds on your back. Calves are what I'd call an aerobic muscle. They are built for endurance; that is why they like high repetition sets to failure ,but with a lot of intensity and weight.

PECS

The best exercises in my opinion are various pressing movements. Cables and flyes are worthless for mass, but later on do give a nice shape to your pecs. I will put my foot down and say that more than 5 sets total is overtraining.

Rules:

1) Always do full repetitions
2) Lower the weights slowly, pause and explode it back up
3) Flex pecs hard between sets to promote pump
4) Never bounce or severe injury could result
5) Increase weight whenever possible
6) Build a routine based on your pec "problems"

Here is a sample routine that I do:
Decline Presses   185 x 12, 295 x 8, 405 x 6
(lower pecs)
Incline Presses   155 x 10, 295 x 5 reps
(upper pecs)

LATS

The best mass movements are Various rows (bent over). There are two kinds of movements: width and thickness. Pick one for each.

Rules:

1) Always use strict form
2) Add weight whenever possible
3) Think of your arms as hooks, and try to pull with you back.

4) On virtually all lat movements you can and should do peak contraction on each rep.
5) Never do more than 5 sets total or you WILL over train.

Example Routine:

Dumbbell Pullovers-15, 12, 10 reps (Teres Major, minor ,Lats)
T- Bar Rows -10, 6 reps (inner back, lower lats, lat thickness)

ERECTORS

Erectors add power and stability to the whole body. As Arnold once said and I agree; the lower back is the seat of power in man. If your lower back is shot; then you will have problems with rows, overhead presses, squats, etc. Dead lifts, weighted good mornings, and weighted hyperextensions are the best mass movements. Do 4 sets for the Dead lifts, if you do them, and only 2 to 3 sets for the other exercises. Add weight whenever possible. Here is a typical erector routine:

Dead lifts- 135 x 8, 225 x 6, 315 x 4, 405 x 2-4 reps.
Your traps, inner back, erectors, and forearms will explode.

TRAPS

Traps are hard to develop for me. One thing you must realize is they get a lot of indirect stimulation from dead lifts, rows, pulls presses etc. So care must be taken not to over train them. I'd suggest you never do more than 3-4 sets. Pulls, cleans, and shrugs are the best for traps. Here is a typical routine that I do:

Shrugs- 225 x 20, 315 x 15, 405 x 6 reps

DELTS

Best width movement is the one arm lateral, and the best thickness movement is the press behind the neck. Never do more than 3 to 6 sets total (for all 3 heads of the deltoid, not per exercise). Always go to failure, use strict form, and try to generate as much pain as possible; for some reason delts love pain and swell up from intense effort and high reps.

<u>Beginners</u>- do just one exercise like presses, or lateral raises, and change the exercise every few months. Add weight all the time. Try to get strong, but don't get hurt! Ex routine:

Lateral raises - (1 arm at a time) 15, 12, 10 reps

Intermediates-You can now do two exercises for different parts of the deltoid. Here is an example routine:

Press behind the neck-3 sets of 12, 8, 6 reps
Bent over laterals-2 sets of 20, 15 reps

Advanced-At the advanced stage you delts must be complete from all angles, so you can do three exercises, but don't exceed 6 sets total.

Lateral Raises-2 sets of 15, 10 reps
Front bar raises-1 set of 12, 8 reps (gets indirect stimulation from bench presses. Direct work may not even be needed.
Bent over Laterals-2 sets of 15 to 20 reps

TRICEPS

If you ever want your arms to break the 20" barrier; then you must blast your triceps hard. They are after all 2\3 of your arm mass physiologically speaking, or they should be. Blast does not mean do a lot of sets either. The triceps get a lot of indirect effect from all the pressing for chest and shoulders. The best mass movements are dips, Close grip presses, and press downs. Triceps like higher reps, pain strict form, and overload.

Beginners- do one exercise for 3 sets, go to failure, and add weight

Intermediates- do two exercises, 2 sets each

Advanced - do only two exercise; 2 sets each but do them heavier, harder, and with more determination. Also change them frequently to avoid plateaus.

Here is a routine that always packs on beef:

Tricep Press downs- 80 x 20, 150 x 6 reps
Dips –Do 2 sets of 50 x 10, 125 x 6 reps (hang additional weight on you with a dipping belt).

BICEPS

Important principles are strict form. Pain, overload, under training, full reps, and stretching movements. The best mass movements are barbell curls, incline dumbbell curls, preacher curls, and weighted chins. Never do more than 4 sets total. That is 2 exercises; 2 sets each. Here is an excellent mass routine I like:

Barbell Curls   115 x 15 reps, 205 x 6 reps
Close grip chins   50 x 8 reps, 95 x 4-6 reps (extra weight). Also if you do this routine, you may not even need to do any direct lat work.

Another routine I like is:

One Arm Dumbbell Preacher Curls-40 x 20, 85 x 6 reps+ partials

Close Grip Barbell Curls- 115 x 10, 185 x 6 reps (cheating)

<u>Beginners</u>- do only one exercise; 3 sets, high reps to failure, and add weight whenever possible

<u>Intermediates</u>- do 2 exercises, 2 sets each

<u>Advanced</u>-do 2 exercises 2 sets each. Just because you are advanced doesn't mean more sets is the prerequisite for growth.

By this time you should be a lot stronger, and able to generate more mental intensity into each rep, and set.

FOREARMS

Forearms should be worked hard unless yours are growing just from gripping. My do grow just from gripping; like if I'm doing 500lb dead lifts; otherwise I do 4 direct sets for them. 2 sets for the flexors, and 2 sets for the extensors. I never do any direct work for the Brachioradialis, as they get worked in all rowing, and lat pulling exercises. Forearms are stubborn and respond better from 100 lbs for 20 reps than doing 200lbs for 6 reps. Add weight when possible and do as many partials as possible after full reps are no longer possible. Here is an example forearm routine:

Wrist Curls- 95 x 30 reps, 150 x 15 reps + partials (10-20?)
Reverse Wrist Curls 45 x 25 reps , 95 x 20 reps

BEGINNER, INTERMEDIATE , AND ADVANCED ROUTINES

Fact: the bigger you get; the more stress a working muscle puts on your recuperative powers. As you get bigger, you will need more and more rest time between workouts. Your strength can double or triple, but your recuperative powers really never improve. If you over train your biceps they might be sore for 4 or 5 days. Furthermore, the physiological processes that allow for growth won't be dictated by man's ignorant routines. Your schedule may say to work them again on Thursday, but they aren't going to hurry up and recuperate because you think you have to train them again so soon. Recuperative processes can't be rushed. Your body must do what it has to do, at its own pace, and that could take 2, 3, or even 5-7 days.

Something that makes me sick is that all magazines say you are a beginner the first month- 1 year and intermediates 6 months- 1.5 years depending on where you read it. They also say you are advanced after 1 or maybe 1.5 to 2 years. That makes me sick! So, if you train for 6 years, but have 14 " arms that makes you advanced? Not in my book you aren't! To me your size dictates level of advancement. For example, if you have:

12 to 15" arms you're a beginner
15 to 16" arms you're a beginning intermediate
16 to 17" arms you're a intermediate
17 to 18" you're advanced intermediate
19 to 20" you're advanced
If your arms are 21 or more inches you are Somewhere On The Other Side Of Huge.

The reason I told you all this is in the pages to come, there are many routines. You must pick the one that is appropriate for your level of development.

Here is the best way to split your body up:

Workout A: Legs\Back\Biceps\Forearms
Workout B: Calves\Chest\Shoulders\Triceps

Exception - Beginners do the whole body 2 times a week for 6 months to a year. Split routines aren't a sign of advancement at this stage, but are a shortcut to disaster.

Examples of beginner routines:

Squats	3 sets	Thighs
Leg Curls	3 sets	Hamstrings
Rows	3 sets	lats, ribcage

Bench Press	3 sets	pecs
Military presses	3 sets	delts
Barbell Curls	2 sets	biceps
Dips	2 sets	triceps
Wrist curls	2 sets	forearms

or

Leg Press	3-4 sets	Thighs
Stiff Leg Dead lifts	2 sets	Hamstrings
1 Arm Db Rows	3 sets	Lats
Db Bench Press	3 sets	Pecs
Military Press	3 sets	Delts
Incline Db Curls	2 sets	Biceps
Lying Triceps ext	2 sets	Triceps
Standing Wrist Curls	2 sets	Forearms

Beginners do this routine 2 times a week like on Monday and Friday, or Wednesday and Sunday

Rules:

1) Add weight whenever possible.
2) Adhere to strict for on all movements.
3) Flex all muscles in between sets.
4) Change exercises every 2 to 3 months.

Beginners- work the whole body twice a week as follows:

Days	Mon	Tues	Wed	Thurs	Fri	Sat	Sun
Workout	X			X			

For all the following levels of advancement; please use the following split: do the traditional leg/back/bicep + chest/shoulder/tricep routine.

Workout A-Leg/back/biceps/forearms
Workout B-chest/shoulder/tricep

Here are some examples of a typical Leg/back/bicep and chest/shoulder/tricep split:

Workout A

Squats	4 sets	Thighs
Leg Curls	2 sets	Hamstrings
Pullovers	2 sets	Lats, Serratus
Rows	3 sets	Lats
Deadlifts	4 sets	Erectors, Traps
Barbell Curls	2 sets	Biceps
Incline Curls	2 sets	Upper Biceps
Wrist Curls	2 sets	Forearms

Workout B

Standing Calves	3 sets	Gastrocnemius
Bench Press	3 sets	Pec, Delt, Tricep
Incline Press	1-2 sets	Upper Pecs
1 Arm Laterals	2 sets	Lateral Delts
Bent Laterals	2 sets	Posterior Delts
Tricep Pressdown	2 sets	Lateral Triceps
Close Grip Bench	2 sets	Rear Triceps

Now these are approximate splits. You may Like Leg Presses better then squats. Fine!

Determine what level you are at, and plug the workout days into the appropriate routine.

Following are tables showing exactly how often you should be working out depending on your size (not years of training).

Beginning Intermediates

Day	Mon	Tues	Wed	Thur	Fri	Sat	Sun
Workout	A	B	Rest	A	B	Rest	rest

Intermediates

Day	Mon	Tues	Wed	Thu	Fri	Sat	Sun
Workout	A	Rest	B	Rest	A	Rest	B

An Advanced Intermediate should follow this regimen:

Day	Mon	Tue	Wed	Thur	Fri	Sat	Sun	Mon	Tue
Workout	A	Rest	B	Rest	A	Rest	Rest	B	rest

Advanced

Day	Mon	Tue	Wed	Thur	Fri	Sat	Sun	Mon	Tue	Wed
Workout	A	Rest	B	Rest	Rest	A	Rest	B	Rest	rest

If you are really Brutally Huge (arms 20 to 21 or more inches); then do this routine:

Day	Mon	Tue	Wed	Thur	Fri	Sat	Sun	Mon	Tue
Workout	A	Rest	Rest	B	Rest	Rest	A	Rest	rest

Remember as you get bigger and more brutally huge, you will need more recovery time. If you really want to grow badly enough, you'll listen to me. You might be saying that there is too much time between workouts. Believe me, you won't shrink! You should be able to take two weeks off and not lose anything. If you do; then I must ask, what kind of muscle mass did you build in the first place? Real muscle takes months to lose an inch.

Here are some rules to aid in recuperation and growth. Every 3 months, take off 1 week to allow for complete recovery of the nervous, endocrine systems, joints, mind, and muscles. Have you ever noticed how thick and energetic and rested you feel after a few days off? Or are you that paranoid that after one day off you imagine your arms will have shrank an inch. Rest equals growth.

Workout A	Sets	Muscle affected
Squats	4 sets	thighs
Leg Curls	3 sets	hamstrings
Pullovers	3 sets	Lats, Serratus
Rows	3 sets	Lats
Deadlifts	4 sets	Erectors, Traps
Barbell Curls	2 sets	Biceps
Incline Curls	2 sets	Upper Biceps
Wrist Curls	3 sets	Forearms

Workout B

Exercise	Sets	Target
Standing Calves	3 sets	Gastrocnemius
Bench Press	3 sets	Pecs, Triceps
Incline Press	3 sets	Upper Pecs
1 Arm Laterals	3 sets	Lateral Delts
Bent Laterals	3 sets	Posterior Delts
Triceps Pressdowns	2 sets	Lateral Triceps
Close Grip Benches	2 sets	Rear Triceps

Now these are approximate splits. You may Like Leg Presses better then squats. Fine! Determine what level you are at, and plug the workout days into the appropriate routine. The most important principle I must pound into you is that of resting as long as it takes to heal and grow. This is the most difficult of all techniques to grasp. A lot of growth comes from just sitting there, eating and resting. Conquer this one difficult way of thinking and unlimited size is yours.

WHEN HUGE IS NOT ENOUGH

This course will show you how to smash through puny barriers like the 16 to 18 inch arm. It will show you how to get out of plateaus and ruts. When Huge is not Enough is a very specialized course, henceforth it is very concise and to the point. The course is not really for the beginner who is just starting out, has 14 inch arms, and is not satisfied with his 1/4" a month gains. This course is for bodybuilders who have been training for years, and whose arms for example have been stuck at 16, 17, or 18 inches for 6 months, 1 year, or maybe even longer. I myself was once stuck at a plateau for 1 year and 3 months. My arms were stuck at 18", and no matter what I did for them, no matter how hard I trained, they would not grow. Intensity techniques, more protein, more weight, forced reps, and nothing else would make my arms grow, or any body part for that matter. It was at that point that I did 2 things. It was then that I started formulating the Brutally Huge System. The other thing I did before I invented the Brutally Huge System was getting real fed up with working out. I started going through all of the usual excuses: moaning and crying about lack of genetics, or it's because I didn't do drugs, or because I wasn't in California; you name it, I made them up. I got so fed up with hopelessness and despair that my arms would forever be a puny 18". So, I decided that I was just going to go on a maintenance workout. That means I'd just work out enough to maintain what I had. At the same time I remember there was this burning desire to work out less often anyway. I was performing the usual 4 day per week routine; doing legs/back/biceps on Monday and Thursday, and doing chest/ shoulders/triceps on Tuesday and Friday. This system worked well enough to get my arms from 15.5 to 18 inches. However as you get bigger your needs do change as I was about to find out.

I mean here is how I was feeling, I would do the leg/back/biceps workout on Monday, and then when I was suppose to come in for Tuesday's workout, I was still feeling burned out, my nerves were shot, my body ached, my joints ached, and my attitude was lousy. Oh jeez I thought to myself, I have to do this stupid workout! It wasn't so much a matter of my legs/back/ biceps being sore as it was my whole nervous system, and recuperative subsystems which needed the rest. I wasn't resting long enough between workouts, and I knew it. I was burned out. How I dreaded coming in on that Tuesday or Friday.

Your average bodybuilder thinks that if he works his legs on Monday and his chest on Tuesday that his legs are recuperating! Right? Wrong!!!! You see when you work your legs on Monday; on Tuesday your recuperative systems are trying to repair the damage, and recuperate your legs. That takes lots of energy.

When you work your chest on Tuesday that also takes energy. Guess where that energy comes from? The energy you used up on Tuesday's workout could've been going towards recuperation from Monday's workout! No human body has two separate banks of energy, one to work out on, and the other to grow on. How ignorant!!!!!! You have only got so much energy, and everything you do saps more of it from you. I hope you are not so misinformed so as to think that your body has unlimited energy and that it'll grow from whatever gross workloads you may impose on it. Your body doesn't care about your little workouts that are religious in nature. If you severely tear down a lot of leg mass on Monday; then it just might take 4 or 5 days to recuperate it, and your body doesn't care about what some ignorant workout doctrine says that you have to work them out on Thursday. I'm telling you most bodybuilders are very fixed in their ways, almost to the point of being resistant to changes that might be beneficial. You might be saying: "yeah but if I don't work them on Thursday again they'll start shrinking"! Well I say how can they start shrinking when they are still sore form Monday and they are still trying to recuperate and grow? Think about this for a moment!!!!

The key to growing is to acquire more energy than you expend. Fact: your recuperative powers really never improve at all, so taking that into consideration; if it took 3 days for your 14" arm to recuperate from a workout; then how much longer would it take a 20", or even a 23" arm to recuperate, assuming your recuperative powers stay constant. However, in real life, those same recuperative powers get worse with age. I'll bet you didn't know that some of the most massive bodybuilders only work a body part once every 5 to 7 days in the off season when they are trying to get even bigger? Did you? Do you really believe that they are working out 3 times a day to get bigger? Obviously, since recuperative rates don't hurry themselves, then the time between workouts must be increased, since there may be a 1/2 foot more of arm size to recuperate. So, as you get bigger you must train less often. That is part of the foundation of the Brutally Huge System. You must adhere to this simple principle if you ever wish to get huge without drugs. It is very important that you understand the concept of under training and the avoidance of overtraining. As long as you over train you will never grow....period!!!! You can waste your money on all the supplements you want, or drugs and you still won't grow. Eating too much will only make you fat. Drugs will pump your over trained little muscles full of sodium and water, so when you go off them and lose all that water; then you will be smaller than before, because you were overtraining all along and destroying real tissue, while you were pumping them full of water.

If you knew the exact number of sets, then you could grow at the optimal or fastest rate possible. With the exception of me and a few other people; how many of you know the exact number of sets? One thing is for sure; that if you over train you will never grow, you might even shrink! However if you were to under train; you might not grow as fast as you could at an optimal rate, but you would always grow. A 1/8" a month on your arms is a small gain but in 12 months that would come out to 1.5 inches; that's not small. Furthermore in 5 years your arms would be 7.5 inches bigger. Think about it!

You might be asking... so where does all of this come in? Your arms, legs, or nothing else for that matter have grown in 8 months or 1.5 years. You're fed up, ready to throw in the towel, and blame it on poor genetics, and now you've justified the need for drugs! However as a last resort you thought you'd order this course and give it a try. Well I hate to glorify myself, but this is your lucky day! Because I just happen to know what your problem is. Remember when you were a rank beginner, and how sore you were after your first workout after a lifetime layoff? You grew like a maniac. That's because it was new to your body. When you are in a rut the worst thing you can do is more sets, more ultra-intensity, 20 sets per body part to supposedly shock them, or training a muscle 3 days in a row. In my opinion, this is just plain ignorant thinking! All of the above techniques will only push you into a farther state of overtraining. At this point the best and only thing to do is take 1 full week off from the weights. Do not just take off two days, not four days, I mean one full week; no less than a week, preferably more if you've got the guts to. No need to worry because you can't train for a week. You've got your whole life to lift the weights. Let's face it, you aren't growing, and deep down inside you are sick of it anyway. Besides if you are so afraid of not training for a week because you might lose a precious little 1/4" of your little, over trained arms; then I must pose this question, what kind of muscle did you build in the first place? There are more important things in life and in the universe than your measurements or mine for that matter. Also, if you are that afraid of a layoff; then it just goes to show how neurotic about training you might be. All of which just further proves the need for a layoff.

Training should be fun and profitable in terms of muscle gains. So take one week off, enjoy life, and have some fun, and don't go to the gym just to hang out either. Eat whatever you want, put on a little weight, and quit being neurotic about your cuts. No one in the world cares about a vein on your belly except you!!!

You need to relax and recuperate mentally and physically. Take one week off, got it??? Now when you come back you need a whole new approach to training. One that'll stimulate growth, yet not be so taxing on your nerves that you can't grow. Your nerves and your adrenal cortex are more important than your muscles. I have determined that the best split is to do legs/back/biceps on one workout and do chest/shoulders/triceps on the other workout. If any of you are complaining that after doing legs that you are too burned out, that is because you were doing 8 to 25 sets for them. That would kill anyone, or your cardiovascular system might be in poor shape. A little bit of cardio, 2 or 3 times a week is all you need for excellent cardiovascular conditioning, and believe me squats won't tire you anymore. Now we must determine guidelines for levels of advancement. To me size indicates levels of advancement not years of training under your belt. I don't care if you've been training for 10 years, if you have 14" arms, then you are a beginner. You don't know anything about proper training; if you did you would have 22" arms by now. So here are some tentative guidelines:

Level	Arm size
Beginner	10-15 inches
Intermediate	15-16 inches
Advanced int.	16-18 inches
Advanced	18-20 inches
Beyond huge	21 or more inches

Now I know this book is supposed to be for advanced people who are stuck in a rut, However, I included a complete review of all levels of experience and how you should train at that level.

Actual routines are listed below:

Beginners- Do a whole body workout twice in 7-8 days. Do about 6 basic exercises, 2-3 sets each of Squats, Bent Rows, Bench Press, Shoulder Press, Barbell Curls, Tricep pressdowns, Standing calves and sit-ups.

Day	Mon	Tue	Wed	Thur	Fri	Sat	Sun
Workout	X			X			

Beginning Intermediates do this split:

Workout A-legs/back/biceps
Workout B -chest/shoulders/triceps

Perform the 4 day a week split on these days:

Day	Mon	Tue	Wed	Thur	Fri	Sat	Sun
Workout	A	B	Rest	A	B	Rest	rest

Intermediates

Day	Mon	Tues	Wed	Thur	Fri	Sat	Sun	Mon
Workout	A	Rest	B	Rest	A	Rest	B	rest

Advanced Intermediates

Day	Mon	Tues	Wed	Thur	Fri	Sat	Sun	Mon	Tue	Wed
Workout	A	Rest	B	Rest	A	Rest	Rest	B	Rest	A

Advanced

Day	Mon	Tues	Wed	Thur	Fri	Sat	Sun	Mon	Tues	Wed
Workout	A	Rest	B	Rest	Rest	A	Rest	B	Rest	Rest

Beyond Huge

Day	Mon	Tues	Wed	Thur	Fri	Sat	Sun	Mon	Tues
Workout	A	Rest	Rest	B	Rest	Rest	A	Rest	Rest

Beyond Huge, plateaued, under stress, over 35-40 years of age

Day	Mon	Tues	Wed	Thurs	Fri	Sat	Sun	Mon
Workout	A	Rest	Rest	Rest	B	Rest	Rest	Rest

Below are the general guidelines for the number of sets that are allowed. Beginners just do 1 exercise for 3 sets each. Everyone else do what is listed below.

<u>Thighs</u>- do 4 sets
<u>Hamstrings</u>-do 2 sets
<u>Calves</u>-do 2 sets
<u>Chest</u>-1st exercise do 3 sets, 2nd do 2 sets
<u>Back</u>- 1st exercise do 3sets, 2nd do 2 sets
<u>Shoulders</u>-2 sets for side, and 2 sets rear delts
<u>Triceps</u>- do 2 exercise for 2 sets each one
<u>Biceps</u>- do 2 exercise for 2 sets for each one
<u>Forearms</u>-2 sets of reverse curls, and wrist curls

If you are at the level of Beyond Huge; then you are an exception to the rule, follow these guidelines:

<u>Thighs</u>-4 sets or 2 supersets like leg extensions and squats

<u>Hamstrings</u>- do 2 sets
<u>Calves</u>- do 2 sets
<u>Chest</u>- do 3 sets of the 1st exercise, 2 sets of the 2nd)
<u>Back</u>-do 3 sets of one exercise
<u>Delts</u>-do 3 exercises, 2 sets each deltoid head
<u>Triceps</u>-do 2 exercises 2 sets each exercise
<u>Biceps</u>-do 1 exercise 2 sets
<u>Forearms</u>-do 2 sets of wrist curls, 2 sets of reverse wrist curls

At the Beyond Huge Level, The biggest and most important concept is that of resting longer and longer between workouts as you get bigger. Another big exception is that now you should be changing the exercises every 2nd or 3rd workout. This is the confusion principle, and I don't really intend for it to be used as a confusion shock technique. If you've noticed you are doing an awfully low number of sets, which is the greatest thing on Earth for mass, but isn't so great for shape. In my opinion shape is largely genetic, but if you do a low number of sets in a workout; the only way to hit the muscle from all angles is to change the exercises very often. Make sure you are consuming a sufficient number of calories each day. You'll know if you are, by observing if you are gaining or losing weight. Also make sure your protein intake is high enough, about 1gram of protein for each kilogram you weigh. When using this principle, as the intensity goes up so does the damage to the muscle, and therefore the protein must go up. Drink more water when you consume more protein as it is beneficial to your kidneys. Too much protein can strain them, and water flushes them out. Be sure to take a good multivitamin/multimineral tablet once each day and add extra vitamin C each day to prevent getting run down and sick. Follow all of the information contained in this course and you will grow. Get Huge!

ICH THIGHS AND 20 INCH COWS

This course will outline in very graphic detail what it takes to get your thighs huge fast. 30" is what my thighs happen to measure. I am 5' 11.5". However, if you are 5'5"; then a 27" thigh will look like 30", and if you are 6'2"; then you will need a 32" thigh to look in the same proportions as me, or the guy who is 5'5".

Many bodybuilders skip or neglect their legs. They are only concerned with working the showier chest and arm muscles. Although I myself love having large arms, I don't neglect my leg training. Nothing looks more ridiculous than someone who has 20" arms and 22" thighs. It is almost grotesque and comical. Furthermore, we all know that heavy leg work has an indirect effect on the growth of the whole body. So, I don't see how anyone could get a 20" arm anyway unless they had blasted their thighs, and trained their torso hard at the same time. We are getting off track though, as this is supposed to be a thigh and calf course, not an arm course. However, I just wanted to point out the benefits of heavy leg training. I mean if you did put on 4" on your thighs and your bodyweight went up 15 to 20 lbs; then don't be surprised if your arms also correspondingly grow 1 to 2". This is as long as you are simultaneously working your arms hard too. So, now we have another good excuse as to why we should do hard leg work: bigger arms. We can't beat that deal, can we? To sum it up, if you ever want your whole body to get huge; then you will have to blast your legs for all you are worth, and that doesn't mean overtraining them and doing an enormous amount of sets either.

Getting to the point, the best thigh exercise in the world is the squat, or more correctly full squats. In the beginning I was one of those top heavy bodybuilders who never worked legs. My justification for not training legs was that squats built a big butt, and that since I trained at home and I didn't have a squat rack to do heavy squats, then I couldn't do legs. What a bunch of silly excuses! It is a good thing I smartened up fast. I also figured that since I didn't have any leg extensions, or leg press machines that was all the more reason not to worry about legs.

At Home Trainers

At home, however, you can still do barbell hack squats. Now that I have told you this and now that I am going to tell you how to do them, you have no excuse not to do leg work if you train at home. Simply put a loaded barbell on the floor, stand in front of it and while looking straight ahead; squat down and grab the bar, and then just stand erect. Also, as an added benefit, this exercise also has an indirect effect on the forearms since all that weight is dangling there they must work hard to hold on to it for a full set. All you need to do is 3 or 4 sets, and try to keep your back straight, use slow strict form, and increase the weight whenever you can. So...... if you workout at home you have no excuse not to train your thighs or hamstrings either. For hamstrings you can always do 3 sets of weighted good mornings or stiff leg deadlifts. I personally think that stiff leg deadlifts and weighted good mornings work the hamstrings better than traditional leg curls.

A sample leg workout at home might be:
Barbell Hack Squats-3 sets of 15, 10, 6 reps
Stiff leg Deadlifts-3 sets of 10, 8, 6 reps

Home trainers can also find ways to improvise and train your thighs hard. Another alternative is that you can do Sissy squats with a weight belt around your waist. Do these in a door way and just hold onto the door jambs for balance. Three sets should be sufficient.

Yet another exercise you can perform is the one legged squat, once again do it between two door jambs and hold on for balance.

One legged squats can feel stressful on the knee ligaments I have found, so do them very slowly. Make sure your foot is close to where it would be as if you were doing 2 legged squats. Once again, 3 sets should be sufficient. Use a weight belt when you are strong enough to do so.

Lastly, they make (and I own one) these hip harness belts that are capable of holding around 400 lbs of plates, or even a bar, and you can put your hands at your hips, and squat without any weight on your shoulders.

Squats are the number 1 mass builder. Nothing builds mass as fast as these. Leg Presses are the second best alternative and hack squats are a distant third choice. Like I said earlier I started doing barbell hack squats at home. When I first started doing them my thighs were a puny 19.75". That was in August of 1979, but 6 months later they were 24". I put 4.25 " on my thighs in a 1\2 year. Now I'll be the first to admit that part of the reason for this massive growth was the fact that I had never worked them before in my life, so it was an initial spurt of growth. When I later started working out at a public gym, I now had access to a leg curl machine. Due to hamstring growth my thighs now measured 25". By August, a year later they now measured 25.5" That is a gain of 5.75" in one year.

I didn't experience any explosive growth until I started doing barbell full squats. My thighs had been stuck at 25.5" for a year and experiencing no growth at all! Then; I started working out at a gym in Manhattan Kansas, and a powerlifter, who is now world class, got me into doing heavy full squats, dead lifts, and other basic movements. Heavy full squats were such a shock that my thighs grew 3\4 of an inch in the first month. When I first started doing squats; the most I could full squat was about 185 x 4 reps. Within a few months I was squatting 315 x 2 parallel reps, and could go all the way down with 295 for a couple of reps. I thought, and still do think that it was quite an improvement for someone who has never squatted before. I remember around New Years of 1981; I became a "basic movement" freak, meaning that if you couldn't use a barbell; then I didn't do the exercise. I just wanted to use barbells and handle the heaviest weight that I could, and get Brutally Huge! All I did was barbell exercises, i.e. Squats, rows, dead lifts, curls, bench presses, etc. All I did was basic movements, with as much weight as possible, and believe me I was constantly pushing the weights up. I was eating nonstop because I was so hungry from those heavy basic workouts. I went from 195 to 225 lbs in about a half year. My thighs were growing anywhere from 3\4" to 1.25" every month for 4 to 5 months nonstop. Here is the exact routine that I did for 6 months:

Squats: 135 x 25, 205 x 15, 295 x 12, 385 x 4 reps. Now of course this was the weight I could do at the end of 6 months. I remember at the time that I could full squat 415 lbs. for a rep. For hamstrings I was doing 3 sets with the same weight:

Leg Curls-3 sets of 15 - 20 reps with about 80 lbs.

Initially in those early days, here is the way I did squats. I always used a board under my feet. Squatting flat footed seemed to use more gluteus and erector than pure thigh power. When you squat with a board under your heels it shifts the stress more down to your middle and lower thighs. I also kept my feet fairly wide; about 1 to 2 feet apart. This strongly stresses the inner thighs. At one time my inner thighs were getting so huge; that my thighs were rubbing together whenever I walked, and it was causing heat and friction that was burning holes on the insides of my pants. At any rate, I digress, back to the bit about stance width.

When you put your feet real close together you will stress the outer thighs. When your feet are far apart, you will stress the inner thighs. I'd put the bar right across my bunched up traps; this (the traps) would provide a cushion for the bar to rest on. You don't want the bar rest on the one large cervical bone that is sticking out of the lower rear portion of your neck. With the bar on my traps, head up, feet apart, I would take in a very deep breath and slowly lower down as far as I could go. As a matter of fact, I would and still do the movement in an exaggeratingly slow fashion. After all, if you don't bounce at the bottom, you can't get hurt. Once I hit bottom I'd explode upwards as hard as I could. On the way down I would concentrate on feeling the thigh tightening up in resistance to what I was doing. I would feel the burn.

Full squats will usually never hurt you if you 1) warm-up properly, 2) never bounce , and 3) descend very slowly in the correct groove, and don't have any knee issues/injuries in the first place. What I have found to be a good warm-up set for your thighs is 1 or 2 sets of 25-50 reps on the leg extension with a light weight, about 60 lbs will do. Nothing heavy! When I was trying to get really huge I wasn't rushing in between sets. Those 4 sets that I would do for my thighs would sometimes take 1\2 hour to complete. I found myself sometimes taking 10 minutes between the heaviest sets. I guess back then, I felt it took that long for me to get physically and mentally prepared for the next heavy set. Now though I usually get those same for sets done in 10 to 15 minutes. After years of squatting my cardiovascular system has gotten in much better shape. Now squats don't usually put me out of breathe unless I do a set of 100 reps. If you want to get the maximum number of reps out of each set; then you must rest a long time in between those sets. There is nothing wrong with taking 5-7 minute rests between sets, if that is what you need, so that you can fully do justice to the next set. If you are still breathing hard from the last set, then how are you going to do justice to the next set?

If you pressed me for the one technique that I feel would make this course worth your money, and that would make your thighs grow fast it would be this:

Intensity of effort at the moment of failure.

What I mean is, you must go to failure and you must go to the point where no matter how hard you try; you get stuck in the middle of the squat. And stuck you must get if you want your thighs to grow an inch in one month. You must go to the point where you know you are going to get stuck, but you give it all you've got anyway. Always have two spotters ready to get the bar off you. It is this kind of extreme effort that will blast size on fast. Now the minute you get stuck in the middle of that impossible rep; don't have the spotters get the weight off you. Let yourself sink all the way down; resisting it all the way. Now don't sit down there but do resist it down and then have them save you and/or help you back up, sort of performing a forced rep, if you will. Try to add 5 lbs per workout on the last sets. If you don't do all of these techniques then don't come screaming to me because you didn't put a 1" on your thighs! Some people might be able to add 1.5", and some might only add a 1\2". Everyone is different. I happened to put an inch on every month for about 5 months. Believe me; I was hungry for brutal size. You have to be that driven, to grow like that.

Hamstrings are simple: just do 3 sets of high reps, and go to failure. Do slow and controlled movements. Here is an example routine:

Leg Curls 50 x 20, 70 x 15, 80 x 12 reps. Add weight whenever you can get the required number of reps. Change the exercises whenever you are sick of them, or they no longer produce results.

Never do more than 4 sets for the thighs, and never do more than 3 sets for the hamstrings. If you do, then you won't grow, especially if you are like most people, namely a hard gainer. So when you think that 1 or 2 extra sets won't hurt, and you don't grow as a result of adding those extra sets, then don't come crying to me. Please follow the advice outlined in this course. Three sets is usually not enough (as you need sufficient warm-up for the delicate knee ligaments and cartilage), and 5 is too many, I have found. This was derived from years of experimentation and empirical evidence. Why are most bodybuilders so intransigent, that is resistant to change, and afraid to try something new? They all believe you need lots of sets to get huge. Just because the Olympians do lots of sets doesn't mean you need lots of sets to grow. They just happen to do lots of sets because they are on so many drugs, that they can over train, and still bloat up in size. Quite honestly, I hate "coaching" people in person because I'm sick of arguing the point. That is why I have these courses out. They can explain in much better detail than I could. Do you want to grow or not? Then please follow the advice contained in these pages! Assuming that you are working your thighs 2 times a week; then this is an example of how you would be progressing. This is based on a current 315 maximum.

Workout#1-135 x 20, 185 x 15, 225 x 12, 275 x 4-6 reps
Workout#2-135 x 20, 185 x 15, 225 x 12. 280 x 4-6 reps
Workout#3-135 x 20, 190 x 15, 230 x 12, 285 x 4-6 reps
Workout#4-135 x 20, 195 x 15, 230 x 12, 290 x 4-6 reps
Workout#5-135 x 20, 200 x 15, 235 x 12, 295 x 4-6 reps
Workout#6-135 x 20, 200 x 15, 240 x 12, 300 x 4-6 reps
workout#7-135 x 20, 205 x 15, 245 x 12, 305 x 4-6 reps
workout#8-135 x 20, 205 x 15, 250 x 12, 310 x 4-6 reps
workout#9-135 x 20, 205 x 15, 255 x 12 , 315 x 4 reps

Note how your old maximum is now your new normal workout weight.

I would like to add in, as it was not in the original 30 inch Thigh course, a technique that got my thighs incredibly HUGE! It was the year 1989, and I was stuck at a plateau. I started craving the idea of doing squats flat footed. Not mentioned above, I had discovered that squatting with your heels on a 1 inch thick board shifts a lot of the stress to your knee bone (patella) and patellar tendons. I got a bad case of tendonitis in 1981 from squatting exclusively with a board. Also as indirectly alluded to and mentioned above, I healed it fairly fast by flushing lots of blood into the joint by doing 2 sets of leg extensions with light weights for about 20 reps each, before doing the squats. At any rate, let us get back to the new technique that helped me explode up to 259lbs, got my thighs well over 30 inches, and I was just "thick as a brick" everywhere. I am not the originator of this idea, but someone introduced me into the concept of heavy and light days. They complemented each other as the light day gave you the endurance to do the heavy day, as well as working a different type of fiber, and the heavy day made the weights feel easy on the light days. After months of doing this, my typical routine looked something like this:

Heavy day-135 x 10, 235 x 8, 345 x 6, 455 x 4 reps.
Light day-135 x 20, 225 x 15, 315 x10, 405 x 8-10 reps.

Notice that I still adhered to a low number of sets, went to failure on the last set whether it was heavy or light, kept strict form, did the movements slowly, rested as long as I needed between sets, and added weight whenever possible. This type of squatting also improves your cardiovascular system, and stimulates the growth of muscle all over your body. The Heavy and light system was a shock that produced a new spurt of growth. So changing the reps, exercises, and training regimens, but sticking with the principles of under training can help you get tremendously HUGE

20" CALVES

Calves are so easy to grow if you would just under train them. Usually, 2 to 3 sets is all you need to make them grow. The best exercise is the standing calf raise, or the toe press on the leg press machine.

Calves respond best to pain and high reps to failure. Strict form is also very important. Full strict reps with 300 lbs will promote more growth than partial bouncing movements with 700 lbs; like the way most misinformed people do them. Bouncing up and down with 700 lbs will just give you a compressed spine and sore ankles. Before, you start any calf training, stretch them out, and make sure the first set is light; so as to thoroughly flush blood into the area, and warm up the Achilles tendon properly. You should be stretching you calves as you go all the way down on each and every rep of the set. Another point that I would like to make is that when you are in the standing calve machine and your whole body is leaning forward; you are just stretching the Achilles tendon. Here is a better way to do standing calf raises. Keep your whole body straight up and down during a set of standing calve raises and you should be leaning slightly back or away from the machine. At the top of each rep, peak contract them hard and hold for a couple of seconds before lowering.

Rules to follow when training calves:

1) Keep your knees locked tight, very tight. As soon as you bend your leg even an inch the soleus comes into play and robs effort from the gastrocnemius.

2) Always look straight ahead, so you keep your spine straight, and the workload is transmitted down to your calves.

3) Keep your whole body leaning slightly back.

4) Go all the way down on each rep to fully activate all the fibers, and to stretch them.

5) Come up all the way on each rep as high as you can and hold this position for 2 to 3 seconds. Feel those calves cramp and tighten up. This cramping effect will peak the calves, and develop the groove under the calf.

6) Do slow partials until failure when full reps are no longer possible.

A secret exercise that I am now going to reveal to you can add 1 inch to your lower leg in one month. Well, that is what it did for me at any rate. These are the reverse of the calf raise or what I call the Tibialis raise. With your heels on the calf board, and your toes hanging off in midair; have someone hold a bar across the top part of your foot, and then you raise the barbell up and down. Increase the weight whenever possible, and you may have to wrap a towel around the bar if it hurts your foot. You can even do this one leg at a time, if you can't find someone to help hold a bar across your feet. That'll make it feel heavier. Working the Tibialis will also cure "shin splints" as well as etch in some detail and mass to the front of your lower legs when they are viewed from the front. The Tibialis can get pretty strong; I am up to where I am using a 135 lb bar for a set of 8 reps. I also believe the tibialis is an endurance muscle and responds better to high reps to failure than low reps to failure. My calves went from 19 to 20.25" in one month using this routine:

Standing Calves	Calves	2 sets 200 x 30, 350 x 15
Seated Calves	Soleus	1 set 400 x 6 (heavy!)
Tibialis Raises	Shins	2 sets 50 x 20, 136 x 6

To work the underlying Peroneus muscles you can stand with your feet on their outsides. That means your whole body weight is on the outer sides of both your feet. You can put a bar on your back or use the standing calve machine. This technique responds best to high reps and really is an excellent therapeutic technique to build flexibility in your ankles especially if you have sprained or injured them before.

Once again, to sum it up for superior calf growth, here are 2 important rules.

Rule # 1-Always keep your knees and thighs locked as hard as you can during a standing calve set. Sometimes your thighs might even be sore the next day from flexing them so hard.

Physiological fact #1-Whenever you bend your knees, even an inch you bring into play the soleus. That is why they invented the seated calve raise.

Can you see the progression of the workload to the soleus? Your whole body should be straight as a board during the standing calve raises. Simultaneously it should also be leaning back too, at a slight angle. You should not be leaning forward into the machine. Something else that is very important. On the standing Calf Raise; putting your feet together works the outer calf, and putting your feet wide apart works the inner calf. Experiment with different toe positions too. Heels in hits the outer calf, and heels out hits the inner calf.

YARD WIDE SHOULDERS AND 22" ARMS

I originally wrote How to get Brutally Huge back in 1987. Since then I have discovered that most people really seem to be hung up on getting their arms as huge as possible. Everything I ever said in How To Get Brutally Huge applies now. The routines and techniques are all the same. Consequently, you will find overlap between the courses, and a lot of the pages even come from the same course. However, there are additional pages you will not find in the Brutally Huge course. This course after all will go into much more detail than the Brutally Huge course, as far as shoulder and arm training goes. This course will show you how to bloat up your deltoids and make your arms look like legs!

Yard Wide Shoulders.... that's pretty wide. The fact of the matter is; maybe I should've called the course How to Look a Yard Wide. First of all, let me say that the only people who are going to get a yard wide are those that are wide naturally, and then through correct training pack on 2 to 4 inches on each deltoid. My own shoulder girth is about 64 1/2 inches and my width is about 29 to 30 inches, and I am wide. However that's how writing goes and people like exciting sounding courses rather than something boring like: "How to Get Bigger Shoulders". A little excitement and hyperbole are very important forms of motivation for the bodybuilder. After all, even if you never bought this course, but if you saw it advertised it would have an effect on your subconscious mind. Even just hearing or seeing the phrase Yard Wide Shoulders will expand your thinking in a positive way. Someone once wrote: anything a man can conceive, and believe; he will achieve. What I'm getting at is this; I don't care how bad you want to get wide, if you don't believe it will happen; then it probably never will. You see the power of the mind is incredible, and the subconscious can't tell between real or imaginary input. Don't even joke about negative things; your mind takes it for real. I have actually gone so far as to put a big sign on my bedroom wall, and it says " BILL DAVIS: 24 INCH ARMS". When you see this every day, it becomes a little more possible for your mind to accept it.

Always tell yourself good things, how big you are going to get; even if you don't yet believe it say it anyway; someday you will. You see there is more to training your shoulders than just doing the same old exercises that everyone else does. It takes something special, it takes every weapon that you have in your arsenal, and the biggest and strongest weapon is your mind. It can make or break your training efforts. Growing is hard enough. You don't need your mind working against you. Put that sign on your wall; a goal that someday is possible to achieve. My arms are 21 inches as of this writing so someday a 24" arm is a reasonable goal, but you won't see me putting an unrealistic sign on the wall like "The 30" Arm. I wouldn't want that, nor could I ever believe it is possible to attain. So, to sum it all, up set realistic goals, and think all the time how you want to look, keep an open and positive mind, and don't relent until you've achieved your goals. Don't ever let anyone tell you it isn't possible; they are just so jealous and insecure they don't want you to succeed. Stay away from "little people" (of course I'm referring to their mentality)

I'd like to touch a little on genetics. First it doesn't matter how wide or narrow you are. You can add an awful lot of width to your existing frame if you just listen to me. If you are already wide then you will get super wide, and somebody who is narrow will get wide; understand? Sometimes desire can make up for genetics. I mean can you imagine how awesome you would look if you were to only put 3 inches on each deltoid in the next couple of years?

Even if you were narrow to start with; you'd look like incredible. There is hope. What I'm about to say is going to upset a lot of you but you're paying me to learn how to get huge; more specifically how to get wide. It is my belief that even if you were to train your shoulders and arms properly, but were overtraining everything else; I don't believe your shoulders and arms would grow at all. I mean if you are overtraining your chest, that may mean you are doing anywhere from 10 to 25 sets total. Well if your chest is getting that much overtraining from all those sets involving pressing movements; then you'd better believe that your delts and arms are getting over trained too. So here is how you should train:

Beginners - do whole body workouts for 6 months to a year

Beginning intermediates, please start a 4 day per week split.

WorkoutA	WorkoutB
Legs	Calves
Back	Chest
Biceps	Shoulders
Forearms	Triceps

Beginning Intermediates- workout 4 times a week on these days:

Days	Mon	Tues	Wed	Thurs	Fri	Sat	Sun
Workout	A	B	Rest	A	B	Rest	rest

<u>Intermediates</u> (arms 16 to 18") keep doing the same split but with added rest days.

Days	Mon	Tues	Wed	Thurs	Fri	Sat	Sun	Mon
Workout	A	Rest	B	Rest	A	Rest	B	rest

<u>Advanced intermediates</u>: follow this regimen

Days	Mon	Tues	Wed	Thurs	Fri	Sat	Sun	Mon	Tues
Workout	A	Rest	B	Rest	A	Rest	Rest	A	Rest

Advanced once your arms are 19 to 20 inches follow this routine:

Days	Mon	Tues	Wed	Thurs	Fri	Sat	Sun	Mon	Tues	Wed
Workout	A	Rest	B	Rest	rest	A	Rest	B	Rest	rest

Once your arms get to around 21 or more inches: then you should go to a routine like this:

Days	Mon	Tues	Wed	Thur	Fri	Sat	Sun	Mon	Tues
Workout	A	Rest	Rest	B	Rest	Rest	A	Rest	Rest

If you are over 35-40 years of age, are already really Huge, under stress, not recuperating well, then do a one day on, 3-4 days off routine. Trust me you will feel better, and that's what part of this game is all about, feeling good!

Days	Mon	Tues	Wed	Thurs	Fri	Sat	Sun	Mon
Workout	A	Rest	Rest	Rest	B	Rest	Rest	Rest

If you really want to get a book size explanation as to why you should train in this manner; then you need to buy "How To Get Brutally Huge". I'm not going to get into it very much here because this section is on shoulders and arms. However, let me say that if you don't rest long enough in between workouts; then you won't grow period! The bigger you are the more you must rest if you want growth to happen. Remember, workouts only stimulate grow, but that growth only happens if you rest long enough for that growth to occur. Most people just workout too frequently, never allow enough time for growth stage to occur. If you really want to grow, then you will do what it takes to grow, even resting more days in between workouts; whether you like it or not. Besides, who the hell wants to lift weights 3 hours a day; every day of the week? If you don't believe me then just keep training the way you are, and your arms will just stay stuck at 16, 17, or 18 inches for the rest of your life. Furthermore, if you think that by just hanging in there that someday growth will happen while in the meantime you go on practicing the same worn out ignorant overtraining methods; then you've got a long wait ahead of you. So before you go and do something dangerous like take steroids because you think you've reached your genetic potential because your arms haven't grown for a year; why don't you try under training for a while? You'd be surprised at how easy it is to grow when you train scientifically. RECUPERATION is the most important thing when it comes to growth. It is more important than diet, exercise, weights, or anything else for that matter, period!

I will go so far as to say this; if you do more than 4-5 sets for your delts; then you just won't see explosive growth, if you see anything at all. Beginners should do just 1 exercise, for 3 sets and add weight every set and as often as possible. Intermediates should do 2 exercises, for 2 sets each; adding weight whenever possible. Advanced trainees should do just 2 exercises most of the time, but sometimes you can do 3, but not for more than 2 to 4 weeks as you will run the risk of overtraining. For example do 3 different exercises; ones which work different heads of the delts. Never do 2 exercises which work the same head in a workout, otherwise you will over train that head. Here is a sample workout:

<u>Press Behind Neck</u>-2 sets 15, 8 reps-side head
<u>Bent Over Laterals</u>-2 sets 15, 15 reps-rear head
<u>Barbell Front Raise</u>-2 sets 20,20 reps-front head

I still say that even if you are advanced; you would be better off sticking with 2 exercises, instead of doing 3 and running the risk of overtraining. The above routine can produce mass if you rest long enough, but it would really be a better routine for pre-contest training, for extra polish, and refinement. When you bought this course, if you thought I was going to tell you some new secret exercise; then guess again. There are no new exercises. But there is knowledge that most people aren't aware of like common sense and avoidance of overtraining. When you are a beginner it is as simple as adding weight, and changing the exercises when they are no longer productive. The same is basically true for the intermediates. However at the advanced stage things get a little more complicated. At the advanced stage I've found that muscles are too strong and adapt to any kind of new routine very rapidly, so staying on a routine for weeks or months is counterproductive. Even if your weights are going up it doesn't mean you will grow. Your tendons and connective tissues can get stronger allowing you to lift more weight even though the muscle won't grow in size.

One of the greatest weapons against stagnation and plateaus is the muscle confusion principle. Whenever you feel even slightly lethargic to the idea of a particular exercise, don't do it. Do an exercise that sounds fun. Do something different. You won't put out the kind of intensity necessary to grow if you have a lousy attitude towards a certain exercise. Workouts must be fun and appeal to you. If you don't look forward to them; then they need to be changed. Variety is indeed the spice of life. Doing a different exercise for your delts each and every workout keeps those delts off guard, and keeps your motivation high; because you will have something new to look forward to. Furthermore, muscle confusion really shocks the delts because they think you are going to do presses again like the last workout, but instead you blast them with lateral raises, and as a result, they are caught off guard.

One very important thing that you must remember to do is keep written records of everything you do so the next time you do a particular exercise you can look it up and see what you did the last time you did it. Since you will only be doing any particular exercise only once; the next time you do it you must do it 5 pounds heavier than the last time you did it. Remember at the advanced stage the Overload principle is still very important. The weight must continue to progress if you want more size. Here is an example of what you must do. Let's say you did press behind the neck on June 1st with 200 lbs for 6 reps; then you did lateral raises on June 6th with 55 lbs for 6 reps; and then on June 11th you do Military presses with 225 lbs for 6 reps. Now let's assume that on the June 17 workout you want to do Press behind the neck; the correct workout poundage would be 205 lbs for 6 reps. If you only get 5 reps then the next time you ever do presses behind the neck again; go for 6 reps, and if you get 7 or 8 reps then the next time you ever do this particular exercise again do 210 lbs for 6 reps. This is a typical progression over a 2 month period. Now I know if you are advanced you will be doing 2 or 3 exercises, but I am only using one for an example. Poundages listed below, are of course for the heaviest set.

June 1st	Press Behind the Neck	200 x 6 reps
June 6th	Lateral Raises	55 x 6 reps
June 11th	Military presses	225 x 6 reps
June 17th	Press Behind the Neck	205 x 6 reps
June 23rd	1 Arm Laterals	35 x 6 reps
June 29th	Barbell Front Raise	50 x 6 reps
July 5th	1 Arm Laterals	40 x 6 reps
July 11th	Military Press	230 x 6 reps
July 18th	Press Behind the Neck	210 x 6 reps
July 24th	Barbell Front Raise	55 x 6 reps
July 30th	Lateral Raises	55 x 9 reps

Can you see how the weights are always progressing slowly? This is what will make you grow; the progressive overload, and the shocking affect of the Confusion principle. Furthermore you will love your workouts because you will look forward to doing them. Many people who use the confusion principle never get any stronger because they always start at the same weight as the last time they did it. Just because you haven't done presses for 3 workouts doesn't mean you got weaker in the pressing movement. Actually you should have gotten stronger from the rest. As long as you are always working out regularly you will never get weaker. Also since you are always doing different exercises you should have more balanced and complete development; henceforth greater overall strength due to all 3 heads being more evenly developed. Can you begin to see the benefits of the confusion principle? Here they are:

1) Better overall shape
2) Shock (from never doing the same thing twice)
3) Enthusiasm and lack of boredom
4) Greater strength
5) And greater SIZE

One word of warning: If you are a beginner or intermediate, don't use this principle. It is my belief that you need to stick with a particular exercise for a month or two, so that you can see the weight you use progress steadily. When you are a beginner or intermediate you're muscles really aren't that stubborn yet; they will respond to very subtle changes in your routines. Changing the exercises once a month or when you are sick of it works better at this stage. At the advanced stage your best weapons are:

1) Muscle Confusion
2) Progressive Overload
3) Visualization
4) Undertraining

One word of caution: no matter what level you are at beginner, intermediate, or advanced; don't go doing 2, 3, or more forced reps at the end of a set, so you can complete more reps. This will only over train you. Only do 1 forced rep on the heaviest set only, and do this only once a week.

SHAPE

At the advanced stage you should be concerned with adding "shapely size", and not just undulated crude mass for the sake of adding mass. Using the delts as example we now know that there is not only the front, side, and rear delts, but there is a lower, middle, and upper section to each delt head. The only way to work all of these areas without overtraining is to use the confusion principle, and change the exercises every month or even every workout, so that over a period of time you are doing all the exercises, and getting even overall development.

PRIORITY

At this point you should be working out the weak muscles first, or the weak areas of a muscle. If you have very overdeveloped frontal deltoids; then you shouldn't be working them more and more, and throwing your front to rear balance out of whack. If you have overdeveloped front delts; then don't do any direct front delt work. The front delts will get plenty of indirect work from your incline presses, and bench presses. Instead, concentrate on working your side and rear delts to balance out the problem. A 20" balanced arm looks a lot better and bigger than a 21" improperly balanced arm, so pay attention to your weak parts. As far as shoulders go, the slope shouldered look is out, so work your rear delts (if you're advanced). As far the actual exercises go; here is a list of a few exercises and the specific areas they work:

The 1 Arm Lateral-Side Delts
Press Behind the Neck-Side, Rear Delts, Traps
Front Press (military)-Anterior Delt
Bent Over Laterals (1 or 2 dumbells)-Rear Delts
Lying on your side Lateral Raise-Lower portion of side delt
Incline Lateral Raise-Rear and rear side delt
Wide Grip rows to the neck-Lower rear delts
Seated Alternate Db Press-Front delts
Barbell Front Raise-Upper front delt

Training to Failure. On all of your specialized delt programs train your weak areas to failure. When full reps are no longer possible; continue on doing the strictest partial reps you can until you can't even do a rep where the weight travels even a mere 2 inches. Don't do jerky partials or you will be robbing the muscle of the benefits. If you are on the pec dec , but turned around so you are working the rear delts; do as many full reps as possible ; as you keep doing reps in strict form you will notice that the range of motion gets shorter and shorter until you can't budge the weight at all in strict form. DO YOU UNDERSTAND THE DIFFERENCE? At the end of a strict set when the weight can't even travel one inch; if you start swinging and jerking the weight wildly of course you'll be able to move the weight 8, 10 , or 15 inches. This however is due to initial torque of a sudden jerk being applied to the weight.

CHEATING PRINCIPLE. The cheating principle is probably the greatest principle you can use when you are a beginner, or advanced for packing on mass, but at the advanced stages all your muscles get so strong that they all "kick in" , and help too much. This only robs the target muscle of the desired effect.

The "smart" Advanced trainees use more deliberate and controlled efforts on all their reps; cheating only to get past the sticking point once or twice at the end of a set. If you really tried hard enough you could probably do 5, 7, or 10 cheat reps on some exercises. Am I saying that you should never cheat? Of course not; just keep it under control. I would say that at this point cheating is only used about 20 to 25 percent of the time.

The Mind of a Muscle. Do muscles do think? Well, probably not. However, people do talk about muscle memory, which implies some sort of a mind like activity, some sort of intelligence. You know, they quit for a year, and come back to lifting, and say, due to muscle memory it'll come back faster the second time. It sounds kind of crazy. If you have done 3 very heavy arms workouts in a row, and all of a sudden you walk into the gym and you feel like doing sets of 20 reps to failure then do it. It could be burn out, or it could be what some people call the intuitive principle. Your real mind, the brain, has ways of knowing what you need. At the advanced stage you've got to listen continually to what your body needs.

At the advanced stage workouts must be fun and interesting. You'll never be able to put forth the kind of intensity needed to grow off a routine that bores the heck out of you, or one that you dread. How many times have you walked into the gym and thought to yourself: "oh no, heavy squats, I don't feel like doing those". To which I say, then don't! Right away, think of something that sounds appealing and do it instead. Variety is indeed the spice of life. Listen to yourself. In the next section you will see the actual routines and exercises needed to build yard wide shoulders and 22" arms. Having all this information at your disposal; what is your excuse for not having 22" arms? I am a pharmacy student, and have taken lots of Anatomy, biochemistry, chemistry, genetics, and physiology classes. I know what I'm talking about. I won't steer you wrong. I want you to get as huge as you can but you must try to eliminate all the other negative garbage from your thinking that you've read, and heard for years. Answer me this: HOW CAN YOU NOT GROW WITH UNDERTRAINING AND EATING A LOT? There is no excuse what-so-ever. So please do exactly what I've outlined in this book and get BRUTALLY HUGE!

HOW TO BUILD A 55" CHEST

This course will show you how I increased my chest measurement from 36 to 55 inches in 9 years. It may take some of you 6 years, and others 12 years; everybody is different. Some of you will never get that big because you follow the ignorant drug based routines of "the champs". Although some top bodybuilders do 15 to 20 sets per body part; even they admit this is only a pre-contest routine when they are on truckloads of anabolic agents and are seeking polish and refinement. I've seen the champs train in the off season, and most of them don't even do half the sets they say they do when they are trying to get huge.

One of the more important things I learned from chest training is the importance of using a full range of motion on all chest movements. You should also change the width of the grip on the chest exercises that involve pressing, so you shock the pec muscles with different grips.

First of all I must stress the importance of under training. As long as you over train you will never grow. I also believe that if you over train your large groups like the legs or back it can throw your whole body into a state of overtraining, and then nothing will grow even if you did train certain muscles correctly.

You read in certain magazines where if you train for 1 year you are advanced just because you've trained that long, but in my book that is all nonsense. Your size dictates your level of advancement. I don't care if you have been training for 10 years if you only have 15 inch arms; then you are a beginner in my book. If you were advanced you'd have the 20 inch arms to show for it. Listed below is a rough guideline to determine where you are; depending on height the numbers may change a little.

Level	Arm size
Beginner	10 to 14 inches
Beginning intermediate	14 to 16 inches
Intermediate	16 to 18 inches
Advanced intermediate	18 to 19 inches
Advanced	19 to 21 inches
Beyond Huge	21 or more inches

The bigger you are the more rest and recuperation that you will need. As long as you continue to over train you will never grow. As I said earlier, if you over train your whole body; then don't expect your chest to grow! All your money on supplements and whatever else will go to waste when you over train. Furthermore, all the pectoral mass in the world won't amount to much if you have a sunken in rib cage. I would say that massive lats and an expanded rib cage account for as much as 75% of your overall chest measurement. If you are a beginner or intermediate, you should be doing one exercise for 3 sets for lats and 2 sets of pullovers for the ribcage. However, don't do 2 lat exercises and 2-3 sets of pullovers, or now you will have done up to 8 sets for lats and 6-7 sets for pecs, which is too many.

Enlarging you ribcage is also very beneficial to the heart, lungs, and other internal organs, as they have more room to breathe sort of and aren't crunched up in a tiny little chest cavity. Also, keep in mind that doing pullovers works your lats, pecs, and rear triceps hard. So adjust your total number of pec, lat, and tricep sets down accordingly, when you are doing pullovers. Here is the best way to expand your rib cage: Do 3 sets of high repetition squats; for instance:

Squats 135 x 25, 225 x 20, 315 x 20 reps

After each set of squats do a set of what I call breathing pullovers. Do high reps, i.e.-15 to 20 per set. After each rep in the squats and pullovers take in 3 deep breaths and hold each one for a couple of seconds. On the pullovers take in the deepest breath possible and slowly let the dumbbell down as far as it'll go. Don't let the air out until you have raised the dumbbell back up. Also as you let the weight down, push outwards with your lungs, as if trying to explode from within, and force your hips down as the weight goes down and they can rise back up as the weight does so that you can take in a deeper breath. If you did your breathing squats and pullovers correctly; then the next day your breastbone will feel tender and sore, kind of stretched out.

Now that we have discussed lat and ribcage training we will discuss the exact methods that will be used to increase the size of your pectoral muscles. If you have naturally large pecs; then I guess you won't need this course. However, since no one knows all there is to know about training, I am sure you will still derive some benefit from this course. Even if your pecs are growing well now they will probably grow better if you under train them. This course will really help the hard gainer. Despite having a 55 inch chest, I have had to go through great pains to increase the size of my chest. One thing you must do is analyze your weaknesses. Below is a list of chest exercises and what area they affect.

Bench press	middle pecs
Incline press	upper pecs
Decline press	lower pecs
Dips	lower pecs

Flat db flyes	outer middle pecs
Incline flyes	upper outer pecs
Decline flyes	lower outer pecs
Decline close grips	lower inner pecs
Incline close grips	inner upper pecs
Pec dec	inner pecs
Cable crossovers	inner pecs
Incline db press	upper pecs
Flat db press	middle pecs
Decline db press	lower pecs

At the beginning and intermediate stages, doing benches is great for overall pec mass. However, at the upper levels the bench is not the "only" chest exercise in the world. Some people never learn this. At the upper stages you must start working on your weak areas. You must start training for shape too. A shapelier chest will make you look bigger too. If your pecs are bottom heavy and sag low; then the last thing you need to do is more decline presses. You should start working on your upper pecs. At the advanced stages you should do 2 movements when training for mass. The first exercise would be to emphasize your weak area, and the second one to hit a different area. As far as shape goes, that'll come from using the confusion principle and changing the exercises every other workout or so to induce variety which will improve shape.

Beginners-should do 1 basic exercise for 3 to 4 sets, add weight whenever possible, train strictly, and change the exercises every 2 or 3 months.

Intermediates-never do more than 5 sets for your pecs, that is 2 exercises; 3 sets for the first one, and 2 sets for the second one. Add weight when possible and be very careful of using too many forced reps or cheating. You should only do one forced rep at the end of the heaviest set for that particular exercise. You will also need to rest more between workouts if you want to grow.

Advanced-the instructions are the same as above, but you will have to rest even longer to grow. Never do more than 5 sets, and at times you will grow better by giving your system a rest by doing just one exercise for 3 sets total. Bringing up your weak points will make you look better and bigger. Forget trying to flatter all the people in the gym with how much you can bench press. You really want to blow people's minds? When they ask you on the street what you can bench just tell them you don't do them. Then they will say something misinformed like: "well, how did you get your arms so big"? Forget benches, all they will give you is a torn pec if you go to heavy, and then you are finished. I'd rather have a 350 pound bench with a 60" chest, than a 500 pound bench with a 50 " chest. The choice is yours. Mass is what counts, and although the stronger you get the bigger you will get, you shouldn't get too hung up on poundage's. Super low reps (like 1, 2, or 3) will not get you huge. If that's all you ever do. Shake things up periodically.

One of the techniques that will help you grow is the saying: "if you can't feel the muscle working; then it isn't". I have found that for me on most pressing movements for the chest; the frontal delts and the triceps perform all the work. Also when you go to heavy on pressing movements you can't feel the weight because you are concentrating too hard on moving it. Also, most people do their presses all wrong; they lower the bar to an area some 2 to 4 inches below their nipples. To better isolate your pecs, the elbows should be kept straight out to the sides, and slowly lower the bar to an area half way between your throat and nipples. Also keep your back flat, don't arch it at all as this shifts the stress to your front delts and triceps. If your pecs aren't pumping up and burning; then they aren't doing the work. Simple!!!!

Another principle that makes your pecs grow faster is what I call the deliberation principle.

Furthermore, the best piece of equipment to use this principle is on the Smith machine. On the Smith machine you don't have to worry about balance. Another technique I discovered, that you will feel in your inner pecs as you do presses on the smith machine, is to keep your back flat, and don't suck in a lot of air. If your chest is too expanded full of air, you reduce the travel distance of the bar. The lower your chest is, the farther down the bar can travel, thus promoting a greater stretch, and henceforth greater development. When you're on the Smith machine doing Benches for example, lower the bar down slowly, let it sit on your chest for 1 to 2 seconds while you build up pec tension (but not enough to move the bar); then explode it up and exhale strongly as you do, so the inner pecs can come into play. Remember you have got to feel those pecs working, pumping and burning.

Here are some sample advanced routine:
Decline Press-3 sets 15, 10, 8 reps
Incline Press-2 sets 10, 6 reps

OR

Incline Presses-3 sets of 15, 12, 10 reps
Dips with weight-2 sets of 10, 6 reps

Change the exercises whenever you are bored with training, or you are no longer getting results from that particular exercise. Remember the keys to getting big pecs are:

1) Undertraining
2) Increased weight
3) Strict Form
4) Variety of Exercises
5) Pain and Pump

Follow these principles and your chest will get huge.

BRUTAL BACK

This course will show you how to pack on slabs of muscle on your back. A weak back will severely limit your progress in other exercises. In my opinion, your back can never get too strong or developed. For instance, if you have lower back problems; then how will you be able to do heavy squats for thigh size, heavy presses for deltoid size, or heavy rows for latissimus development? Furthermore, the 3 exercises I just listed are some of the most important for packing muscle on, all over your body. Leg extensions, cable laterals, and lat pulls just won't do for you what heavy squats, presses, and rows will.

The whole body must be trained properly for any one muscle to grow at a maximal rate. I'm not going to get into the do's and don'ts of my training methods. That is all covered in Brutally Huge and the Body parts. This course is going to get right into back training. Follow the information in these courses and you will grow. There are 4 major areas that we need to concern ourselves with: The inner, lower, outer, and upper back. First we are going to discuss the erectors. Erectors must be developed as thick and as strong as possible, so you won't flat from the side, and so you can safely handle maximum weights in exercises like squats, rows, and overhead presses.

The best exercises for erector mass are:

Deadlifts
Weighted Good Mornings
Weighted Hyperextensions

On the deadlifts you should load up a bar, stand behind it, squat down and grab the bar. The hand that you write with should be in an overhand position, and the other hand should be in an underhand position. Look straight ahead, straighten your back, and stand up erect. As you near the top pull your shoulder blades back, and crunch them together.

Weighted Hyperextensions-Have someone put a 45 pound bar across your shoulders; simply go down to a position of 45 degrees below the parallel, and rise up to where your torso is parallel to the ground. Be careful not to raise up too far and hyperextend your spine. Add weight whenever possible and do only 2 to 3 sets, not 5 or 6 sets, but 2 to 3 sets. No more!

Weighted Good Mornings-Lift a bar off the squat rack like you were going to do squats. Instead of doing the squats lean forward until your torso is almost parallel to the floor. Keep your knees bent slightly, and arch the back upwards as you lower your torso, and when to rise back up. Never let it round out when going up or down. You will also feel this exercise pulling in your hamstrings. Do only 2 sets. No more or you will over train.

On all these exercises beginners should only do 2 to 3 sets. Change the exercises every 2 to 3 months. Add weight whenever possible. Doing more than the prescribed number of sets, will only over train you and result in diminished progress.

Intermediates and Advanced-Same as above but now you should be changing the exercises more often. Use heavier weights, go to failure, and do reps very slowly to better isolate the muscle.

Here is a typical deadlift routine based on a 400 pound maximum:

135 x 8, 205 x 6, 275 x 4, 365 x 2-4 reps

If you would rather do the weighted hyperextensions then do this sort of sequence:

45 x 8, 65 x 6, 85 x 4

Whenever you get the required number of reps; then add 5 more pounds the next workout. Always pyramid your weights, and keep the poundage between sets evenly spaced.

Lats

There are 3 categories here: Width, thickness, and the lower lats. Below are a list of exercises and which area they affect:

Width Exercises	Thickness Exercise	Lower Lats
Front Chins	Barbell Rows	Close grip Rows
Behind Neck Chins	T-Bar Rows	Reverse Grip Chins
Cable Lat Pulls	1 Arm DB rows	Seated Cable Rows
Db Pullovers		
Underhand Chins		
Lat Pulls		

Beginners -when you are this small any exercise will make your lats grow. Just pick one exercise and do 3 sets of it, pyramiding the weights each set. Add weight whenever possible, and use strict form and change the weights every 2 to 3 months. If your torso is 35 to 46 inches, then you are a beginner, and you need more mass before going to an intermediate routine. Adding more sets will only over train you and you will stay small forever. More sets doesn't mean faster growth, it means slower growth, if any growth at all. This I promise you. If you don't believe me; then go ahead and do 20, 30, or 40 sets for your back and see what happens. At that rate you'll never break the 44" barrier.

Here are 2 sample routines for the beginner:

Bent Rows-95 x 10, 115 x 8, 135 x 6
Deadlifts -135 x 8, 165 x 6, 195 x 4, 225 x 2-4 reps

or you can do:

Lat Pulls -100 x 15, 125 x 10, 150 x 8
Weighted Hyperextensions-45 x 8, 55 x 6,65 x 4

Intermediates - If your torso measures 47 or more inches then you are probably an intermediate. Not because you've trained "x" number of years. Size dictates level of placement in my book. Not years of training. At this level, if you want to ever reach advanced size; then the avoidance of overtraining is critical!!!You'll never break the 50" barrier if you over train. Never!!! Pick one exercise for thickness, one for width, and one for the erectors. Do not, I repeat do not do more than 5 sets total for the lats, or they just won't grow, period!!! I mean 5 sets, not 6, or 7, or more. Do you want to grow, or not? Or are you going to follow the crowd, and what you read in magazines and stay small forever? Here are some sample intermediate routines:

Rows	3 sets 15, 10, 6 reps
Lat Pulls	2 sets 10, 6 reps
Deadlifts	3 sets 8, 6, 4 reps

or

T - Bar Rows	3 sets of 10, 8, 6 reps
Weighted Chins	2 sets of 10, 6 reps
Hyperextensions (with added weight)	3 sets of 10, 8, 6 reps

or

Dumbell pullovers	3 sets of 15, 12, 8 reps
Bent over rows	2 sets of 10, 6 reps
Good mornings	3 sets of 10, 8, 6 reps

Always use strict form and add weight whenever possible.

Advanced - If your torso is 50 to 52 or more inches; then you are most likely an advanced trainee. Here is the catch, I have found that as you get bigger it is harder to recuperate, so you must do even less sets or you won't grow. However, to maximize shape training you will use the confusion principle, which means you will be changing the exercises very frequently. Shape will come about as a result of using more exercises, but not in the same workout or you will over train. There is that word again, overtraining. As long as you over train you will never grow. Period! Even the champs who take truckloads of anabolic agents only do that many sets for a short while before a show, and that is to refine, and get more cuts, NOT MASS! This course is how to get big, nothing else. Here are some sample routines:

Bent rows   3 sets of 12, 10, 6 reps
Deadlifts   3 sets of 8, 6, 4 reps

or

T-Bar rows 3 sets of 10, 8, 6 reps
Good Mornings 3 sets of 8, 6, 4 reps

or

Lat Pulls   3 sets of 15, 12, 10 reps
Top Deadlifts   3 sets of 6, 4, 2-4 reps

Here is a sample workout that I did the other day:

Weighted Chinups-1st set: 50 lbs x 10 reps, then 100lbs x 6 reps
Weighted Hyperextensions-45 x 12, 85 x 8, 115 x 6 reps

When you train this heavy you can get pretty sore, and it takes more days to recuperate. Sometimes 3 to 5 days.

The NUMBER 1 cause for no growth is **OVERTRAINING**!!!!!!!!!

The Most important techniques are:

1) Heavy Basics
2) Add Weight
3) Strict form at first then cheating once failure is reached
4) Variety of exercises
5) Proper nutrition
6) Under training

Inner Back

For beginner deadlifts, T-Bar Rows, Squats, and such exercises should thicken up the back adequately. I'm talking about the area right between your shoulder blades. If at the advanced stage you are still shallow there; then obviously you are going to need some specialized training. I have some secret exercises which will pack meat on the area fast. This is one of them:

Find a bench that is about 3 feet high; if you can't; then elevate it up on two concrete blocks so it is high enough. Lie stomach down on the bench with your arms hanging straight down. Grab a barbell off a 6" block of wood or something. Using a 8" grip, shrug the bar straight up and down. As the weight goes down let your shoulders kind of slide forward and let the shoulder blades spread out. You should feel it pulling. At the top of each rep; hold the weight for a count of 2 to 3 seconds.

The other exercise that I like to do is lying on a high bench rows. You assume the same position as in the exercise listed above, but now you row it up with your elbows straight out to the sides, and at the top hold it there for a peak contraction of 2 to 3 seconds. Another great technique I've used is to superset the 2 exercises together: Lying Shrugs with Lying Rows using the same weighted bar. This technique is really good for people who have stubborn inner backs. I am one of those people I should know! 2 supersets is all you should need. Anymore than that, and you will over train. If that doesn't work I have also done Olympic Cleans, and that packs on inner back thickness also, or you can superset Shrugs and Cleans for ultimate inner back development. If you do cleans, make sure you don't do deadlifts that day for your lower back or you will over train the erectors. You could possibly hurt yourself too. Follow all the advice in this course and I know that you too can have a Brutal Back.

Brutal Traps and Delts

First of all, I would like to thank you for buying this course. This course will show you how to pack on slabs of muscle on your Deltoids and Traps. Routines will be provided to bulk up and blast all three heads of the deltoids and the trapezius. I believe that if you follow the instructions to the letter contained in this course; then over a period of time you will get so wide that you won't believe it. First of all, let me clear up this misconception about beginners, intermediates, and advanced trainees: Some magazines say for example that after you have been training for 2 years that automatically makes you advanced. I disagree with that thinking!!! I don't care if you have been training for 10 years. If your arms are 15 inches; then you are still a beginner in my book! Provided below are some rough guidelines to determine what level you are at.

Beginners	arms 10-13 inches
Beginning intermediates	arms 14-16 inches
Intermediates	arms 16-18 inches
Advanced intermediates	arms 18-20 inches
Advanced	arms 20-21 inches
Beyond huge	arms 21 inches or more

Beginners do should do a whole body workout on these days and should probably be doing that whole body workout twice a week.

Days	Mon	Tues	Wed	Thurs	Fri	Sat	Sun
Workout	X			X			

After you are past the beginner stage, here is the split that you should now follow:
Workout A-legs/back/biceps/forearms
Workout B -calves/chest/shoulders/triceps

Here are some example workouts:

Workout A
Squats	4 sets of 10, 8, 6, 4 reps
Leg Curls	2 sets of 15,10 reps
Pullovers	2 sets of 10, 8, 6 reps
Bent Rows	3 sets of 10, 8, 6 reps
Barbell Curls	2 sets of 10, 6 reps
Wrist Curls	2 sets of 20 reps

Workout B
Standing Calves	3 sets of 20, 15, 10 reps
Crunches	2 sets of 10 reps
Decline Press	3 sets of 10, 8, 6 reps
Incline Press	2 sets of 8, 6 reps
Shrugs	2 to 3 sets of 10 to 6 reps
1 arm laterals	2 sets of 15, 8 reps
bent laterals	2 sets of 10, 6 reps
Tricep Pressdown	2 sets of 12, 8 reps

Beginning intermediates do this routine:

Days	Mon	Tues	Wed	Thur	Fri	Sat	Sun
Workout	A	B	Rest	A	B	Rest	rest

Intermediates should workout on these days:

Days	Mon	Tues	Wed	Thur	Fri	Sat	Sun
Workouts	A	Rest	B	Rest	A	Rest	B

Advanced Intermediates should adhere to this regimen:

Days	Mon	Tues	Wed	Thur	Fri	Sat	Sun	Mon	Tues
Workout	A	Rest	B	Rest	A	Rest	Rest	B	Rest

Advanced trainees will of course need even more rest time:

Day	Mon	Tue	Wed	Thur	Fri	Sat	Sun	Mon	Tue	Wed
Workout	A	Rest	B	Rest	Rest	A	Rest	B	Rest	rest

Someone who is Beyond Huge would train in this fashion:

Days	Mon	Tues	Wed	Thur	Fri	Sat	Sun	Mon	Tues
Workout	A	Rest	Rest	B	Rest	Rest	A	Rest	Rest

If you are 35-40 years of age, are Brutally Huge, under stress, not recuperating well, then do a one on, 3-4 days off routine. Trust me you will feel better, and that's what part of this game is all about, feeling good, feeling powerful as well as actually being Huge.

Days	Mon	Tues	Wed	Thurs	Fri	Sat	Sun	Mon
Workout	A	Rest	Rest	Rest	B	Rest	Rest	Rest

Remember, the bigger you get, the more rest time you will need to grow. Although muscles sometimes can recuperate in 72 hours, it's your endocrine system, and all the subsystems that recuperate the muscles that need recuperation. As long as you over train you will never grow! Let us say that you aren't growing now, and you are doing 8 to 12 sets for the Biceps and Triceps; then why don't you try 15 to 20 sets. When that doesn't work try 20 to 30 sets. Keep adding sets until you shrink so much, and are so sick of doing that much work and not growing that you'll quit. Maybe then you will realize that more sets are not the answer, and be more open minded to the concept of doing a super low number of sets. Recuperation is the answer. It truly is amazing.

Do you think your body's growth is rushed or mediated by some man-made routine? If you worked delts on Monday, and the schedule says to do them again on Thursday, but they are still sore, and you train them anyway; then you never let your delts completely heal from one workout before starting the next one.

Growth happens when it is ready to; not because some ignorant routine, which doesn't take into account how the body works, says work delts 3 times a week. That is the main reason there are so few 20" arms, but thousands of little 15" arms. How you ever noticed that all the "champs" propose the same ignorant advice, just do more sets and that'll cure all your problems? I hate to say this, but if you are taking all the drugs they are, then you can get away with it, but I believe someday, you will pay a horrible price.

How to Get Brutally Huge and the Bodyparts goes into extreme detail on working the individual muscles and theory.

TRAPS

Some people's traps grow readily from squats, deadlifts, and overhead pressing movements. These people get sloped shoulder very easily from doing shrugs, upright rows, or anything. I have very stubborn traps which have always been very hard to develop. If you have problems building height to your traps; then I have found that the barbell or db shrugs, done in the following manner can help. The most important technique is what I call a sustained peak tension. If you were doing a set of barbell shrugs you would hold the weight at the top position for a count of 2 to 3 seconds. Shrugging the weight up and down haphazardly is not good enough. Also, don't do what most people do, rolling their shoulders back. That is the easy way out. If you can't shrug the bar up all the way; then don't think you are deriving benefit from the shrugs done in this manner when you are supposed to be shrugging the bar straight up and down. Lighten the bar and strive for full up and down motions. When you roll the shoulders back, you are stimulating the inner back, but not stressing the traps in such a way as to add height to them. To get trap height near the ears you must shrug the bar up as high as possible and hold it there for as long as possible, even 6 to 9 seconds if possible. If trap height is the problem; then I would suggest that you do this routine:

Shrugs (with bar or dumbbells)-3 sets of 15, 12, 8 reps, and hold each rep up as high as possible for as long as possible. Also, try not to go so heavy that you are bending your arms and doing sort of a partial upright row or a pull. You don't have to lock out the arms, but don't start bending them, and consequently stressing your biceps and brachioradialis (upper forearm) more than your traps.

Now if trap tie-ins near the deltoid are your problem area; then cleans and power pulls are the best exercises for you to do. Pulls are just a form of cheating upright rows. With the pulls you just heave the bar to the nipple area, and then let it down slowly. Here is a good workout to stress the tie-ins:

Upright Rows 3 sets of 15, 10, 6 reps

Here is a secret exercise that I have developed for working the traps if you have problems gripping the bar: Go over to the standing calf machine and get your shoulders under the 2 pads, and simply shrug the pads up and down. Also, on each rep make sure that you hold the count for up to 10 seconds if possible.

Deltoids

Beginners- should only do one exercise for 3 sets. Pyramid the weights, and use strict form and add weight whenever possible. Do exercises like the press behind the neck, lateral raises, and military presses.

Intermediates- You can and should do 2 different exercises for 2 different areas. Here is an example routine:

Military presses-2 sets of 10, 6 reps
Bent Laterals-2 sets of 15, 10 reps

Advanced-You can do 3 exercises before a contest, but if it is size you are after; then you should only do 2 exercises. Here is an example of a pre-contest routine

1 arm lateral raises-2 sets of15, 10 reps
Barbell Front raises-2 sets of 20, 15 reps
Bent over laterals-2 sets of 15, 10 reps

I would also like to mention that no matter what level you may be at, if you do lots of incline presses, and bench presses; then your front deltoids are already getting a lot of indirect stimulation, and doing direct sets for the front delts will likely only over train the area.

Here is a list of exercises and what areas are affected:

<u>Front Delts</u>
Barbell or db front raises
Front presses
Alternate front db presses
Cable front raises

<u>Side delts</u>
1 arm laterals
2 arm laterals
Press behind the neck
1 arm laterals with the cable

Rear Delts
Bent over 1 or 2 arm lateral raises
Wide grip rows to the neck
Rear delts on a pec dec machine

Side Delt Tie-ins
1 arm lying on your side lateral raises

Width

   I am not a naturally wide person. I've had to work very hard to get wide over the years. I still feel that to this day the single best exercise for capping off the lateral or side delt, is the 1 arm lateral raise. I presently can do a 1 arm lateral raise with a 125 pound db for 4 reps. In the strict lateral raise I have done 85 pounders for 15 reps. There is a slight cheating motion involved, and you must use this principle to get wide delts. Cheating a little at the beginning of each rep, will allow you to get the heavy weight past the initial sticking point and into the range where the delts can exert full power. No matter what your level of development; the 1 arm lateral is the number 1 width exercise. On all shoulder movements, please make sure the first set has high reps to thoroughly flush the area with blood and warm it up thoroughly. Here is the routine I was doing 2 months ago:

One arm laterals-30 x 20, 75 x 12, 110 x 8 reps
Bent over laterals-30 x 15, 55 x 10 reps

I have learned that the side delts respond best to the 1 arm lateral when cheating is used. You will never get wide doing strict laterals with 20 pound dumbbells. You must cheat only enough to get the weight moving; then power alone must move the weight. It is also advisable to initiate the movement with the dumbbell in front of the thighs. The 2 arm lateral is the next best movement for capping the side delts. You should lean forward about a foot when doing this exercise. Start with the db's in front of your thighs, and raise the db's directly out to the sides. As the db's go up the palms of your hands should be facing straight down. Forget about trying to pour the invisible pitcher of water. That can strain your rotator cuffs. Just lean forward and you will find the palms in the correct position. A lot of people complain about the trap and shoulder blade area cramping when trying to twist their hands; this is because of the rotator cuff muscles working.

For thickness the press behind the neck is probably the best movement that you can do. Standing military presses are a good alternative. The proper way to do the press behind the neck is to lean forward as you press the weight up, and back at the same time. The weight should be slightly behind your head when you are done with the movement. Also, when you press the bar up, force your elbows back as you press it up; this will strongly contract the rear delts too. Some principles that I have learned about delts are:

Delts love the painful workouts, resulting in a severe pump.

Overload and increase the weight whenever possible.

Delt exercises should be done strictly when appropriate.

Don't over train the delts; as they get lots of indirect work from chest and back exercises.

If you over train your delts they will never grow

<u>Beginners</u>-do not ever exceed 3 sets
<u>Intermediates</u>-should never exceed 5 total sets
<u>Advanced trainees</u>-should never exceed 5 sets when training for mass or 6 sets before a show.

Here are some sample routines

<u>Beginners</u>
Routine A-1 arm laterals 3 sets
Routine B-military presses for 3 sets
Routine C-press behind the neck for 3 sets

Intermediates

Routine A
Behind the neck 3 sets
Bent over laterals 2 sets

Routine B
Lateral raises 3 sets
1 arm bent over laterals 2 sets

Routine C
1 arm laterals 3 sets
Front raises 2 sets

Advanced

Same as above, listed below is a precontest routine
Seated Alt Db Press 3 sets
Barbell Front Raises 2 sets
Bent Over Laterals   2 sets

Follow all the advice in this course and your delts will get huge and wide.

HEAVILY ARMED

This book will show you how you can get Brutally Huge Arms. Everybody wants them, but only a few people have them. Why is that? The question requires 2 answers: ignorance and overtraining! Let's face it, there are probably hundreds of little fellows in your gym doing set after set of curls in the mistaken belief that more sets and emulating the illogical routines of the "champs" will give them massive arms. Yet why is it that they all have 12, 14, 15, or maybe 17 inch arms? Once again, the answer is ignorance and overtraining. You will never get huge doing 10, 15, or even 20 sets for your arms. You absolutely never, ever will! If you don't believe me then do 20, 30, or 50 sets for your little arms. When you rip your tendons or lose an inch the first month; then you might believe me! Some of you might be saying: "well who the heck is Bill Davis"? Well there are 2 answers to that! Number one, I have 21" arms and you probably don't; that's why you bought this course, which by the way was the intelligent thing to do, thus giving you a chance to be Brutally Huge, and number two, Joe Weider and Vince Gironda never won the Mr "O", yet you wouldn't dispute the fact that they are probably more knowledgeable than anyone in the world when it comes to muscle growth. Titles don't tell you anything! All they tell you is who was probably taking more drugs. So, by now you should be getting a rough idea of why there are so many little arms in the gym, and only a handful of 18, 19, or 20" arms. The key to getting huge arms is under training, increased stress and overload, and longer rests between workouts. If you did nothing but heavy pressing and rowing movements for your chest and back; your arms would probably grow better than they are now. You must thoroughly convince yourself that more sets are not the answer. Somewhere you've all read some kind of nonsense, in some magazine that you need preacher curls for your lower biceps, incline curls for your upper biceps, and concentration curls for the peak. What a joke! In believing that nonsense and performing it; you will have over trained your arms so badly that they'll never grow. That is another pet peeve of mine. You can do all the concentrations curls you want, but if you weren't born with peak; then no amount of concentration curls will ever give you ever give you a peak! For years I believed that myth, and I never got a peak. My arms just got bigger. Find your strong points and develop them. If you have a 1" gap between your biceps and forearms; then no amount of preacher curls will ever lengthen your biceps. Your lower bicep may get thicker, but that 1 inch gap will still be there. By the way, who started all these stupid myths anyway? If shape training were true; then everybody who has high calves could lower them couldn't they? Learn the facts and ignore the ignorant myths. You are paying me money and I am going to tell you exactly what it takes to grow. If getting big arms was easy, everyone would have them!

One of the biggest myths is that more sets will work more fibers of the muscle. Nothing could be further from the truth! Doing more sets will only over train you. You'll still be sore by the next workout. That's just great; you'll get 20" plus arms real fast over-training like that! Once again, the key to massive arms is under training. That way you will always grow, and there won't be any guesswork. There is one way to tell if you are overtraining. Ask yourself this question: are you growing? If not, then you are overtraining. Don't worry about diet if you aren't losing weight; then obviously you are eating enough. When you under train you can't stop yourself from growing. These courses are full of excellent knowledge and content, and you have spent your hard earned money on them. Taking all of that into account, it would not be prudent to ignore what I have to say. I've taken Physiology, anatomy, Organic chemistry, biochemistry, pharmacology, and nutrition classes; I've trained a lot of people and have performed these and other techniques on all of them and myself for the last 10 years. They work! It is difficult to convince people to change. They won't let go of ignorant training dogma and indoctrination. I am not going to waste your time explaining how to do a barbell curl. We both do the same exercises. It is your attitude, knowledge, thinking, and the way you train that must be changed. Quit groping around in the dark looking for some exercise that'll add 2" of peak. There is no such thing, but if you ever do find it; then let me know because I need more peak also. We've all tried it before you and I can tell you they don't exist!

You ever hear the old cliché "No Pain No Gain"? It is obvious that everybody is going through plenty of pain already from doing 15, 20, or even 25 sets. Here is a better cliché: "the LESS you train, the MORE you gain". Not sure who invented that, but I like it. Master the art of self restraint and you will grow. Leave the gym feeling like you didn't do as much as you wanted to do, and you will grow faster and easier than you previously believed.

You'll never grow doing lots of sets. Never, never, never!!!!!!! Oh, and don't cop out and say you can't grow because you are not taking all the drugs the "champs" do. That is just an excuse to not work hard and smart! Believe in yourself, the contents of this book, and hard intelligent training! You can build 20" arms and keep your health. Forget drugs! Get smart, and you'll get BRUTALLY HUGE! Oh yeah, I forgot, some of you are complaining about having poor genetics.

The fact is that genetics controls things like hair color, height, eye color, skin color, and muscle shape, not size! I know that not everyone can get 24 inch arms, but anyone can get bigger. Even if you only weigh 120 pounds; you can still improve, and weigh 200 pounds years down the road. At any rate, I believe any average person is capable of building at least 17-18" arms. Larry Scott was a skinny kid; however, he eventually developed 20.5" arms, and won the Mr. Olympia. I myself have gone from 140 to 255 lbs, and have put 9" on my arms in 10 years! My arms have gone from 12 to 21 inches. Forget genetics it is a burned out excuse, and I'm tired of hearing it! Finally, you won't really know if you have poor genetics until you've given it everything you've got, including following the advice in this book to the letter.

Once again, the keys to getting huge arms are the following:
Under training

Lots of nutritious food
Heavy basics
Training to failure
Progressive overload
If any of these is missing.....Forgot it!

Levels of placement

In my book your size dictates level of development, not the number of years you have trained. Some magazines say you are advanced after one and a half years of training. The heck you are. That is just to make you feel good. If you have been training for 6 years and still have 14" arms then you are a beginner.

Beginners do whole body workouts on these days, twice a week.

Days	Mon	Tues	Wed	Thurs	Fri	Sat	Sun
Workout	X			X			

After the beginner stage, you can start a split routine. A good split is:

Workout A-Leg/back/biceps/forearms
Workout B-calves/chest/shoulders/triceps

Beginning intermediates (arms 14-17 inches) do this routine:

Days	Mon	Tues	Wed	Thur	Fri	Sat	Sun
Workout	A	B	Rest	A	B	Rest	rest

Intermediates (arms 17-18 inches) should work out on these days:

Days	Mon	Tues	Wed	Thur	Fri	Sat	Sun
Workouts	A	Rest	B	Rest	A	Rest	B

Advanced Intermediates (arms 18-19 inches) should adhere to this regimen:

Days	Mon	Tues	Wed	Thur	Fri	Sat	Sun	Mon	Tues
Workout	A	Rest	B	Rest	A	Rest	Rest	B	Rest

Advanced trainees (19-21 inches) will of course need even more rest time:

Day	Mon	Tue	Wed	Thur	Fri	Sat	Sun	Mon	Tue	Wed
Workout	A	Rest	B	Rest	Rest	A	Rest	B	Rest	rest

Someone who is Beyond Huge (arms over 21 inches) would train in the following fashion:

Days	Mon	Tues	Wed	Thur	Fri	Sat	Sun	Mon	Tues
Workout	A	Rest	Rest	B	Rest	Rest	A	Rest	Rest

If you are 35-40 years of age, are Brutally Huge (have 20-21 inch plus arms), under enormous stress, not recuperating well, then do a one day on, 3-4 days off routine. Follow the routine listed below. Trust me, you will feel much better, and that's what part of this game is all about, feeling good, feeling powerful, as well as actually being Huge.

Days	Mon	Tues	Wed	Thurs	Fri	Sat	Sun	Mon
Workout	A	Rest	Rest	Rest	B	Rest	Rest	Rest

The bigger you get the longer it takes to recuperate. If you don't believe this then you will never get huge! Ever!!!!!!!

Beginners-do 1 exercise for the Biceps, 1 for the triceps. Do 3 sets each, pyramid the weights, go to failure, add weight whenever possible, and change exercises when they are no longer productive perhaps every 1 to 2 months.

Intermediates- same as above

Advanced Intermediates- start doing 2 exercises for triceps and 2 for the biceps. But be careful here as doing two chest movements totaling 5 sets and 2 direct tricep movements, totaling 4 more sets, could add up to 9 sets of combined direct and indirect tricep work, which is way too much. Try to find a way to keep the total amount of set for biceps and triceps down to about 5 sets. It's hard to do, but you will grow better.

Barbell Curls	2 sets of 10, 6 reps
Incline curls	1-2 sets of 8, 6 reps
Lying tricep ext.	2 sets of 20, 15 reps
Weighted Dips	1-2 sets of 10, 6 reps

Advanced - same as above but now you are using much more weight, resting even longer between workouts, and using high intensity principles like cheating, forced reps, etc.

Beyond Huge - Same as above but now you are resting even longer, training even heavier, using the muscle confusion principle, changing the exercises every 2nd or 3rd workouts, and doing slow deliberate movements. Also, make sure you are consuming sufficient calories and a high protein intake i.e. 1 gram of protein for every kilogram you weigh. Listed below are typical arm exercises and what muscle/area they target:

<u>Tricep Exercises</u>	<u>Areas affected</u>
Dips	rear head
Close grip Benches	lower triceps
Tricep Pressdowns	upper side tricep
Lying Ext.	side triceps
Decline Lying Ext.	Upper side triceps
Pullover and extension	rear upper triceps
1 arm ext. across chest	side triceps
1 arm ext beside head	rear tricep

Biceps Exercises	Areas affected
Barbell Curls	overall mass/power
Close Grip Curls	outer biceps
Incline Curls	upper biceps
Preacher Curls	lower biceps
Concentration Curls	peak
Underhand Chins	middle/lower biceps
Hammer Curls	Brachialis
Close Rev.Grip Chins	Biceps/upper forearms

Massive arms don't happen by accident! It takes intelligent training, intensity, placing greater and greater stress on the muscles, and allowing more rest time than ever, to fully recuperate from said stresses. The biggest mistake I see in all bodybuilders who aren't getting the kind of arm results they think they should be getting; is failing to take into account that all back and chest work is already working your arms and is additive in nature. In other words, doing 10 sets for your back and 10 sets for your biceps is a total of 20 sets for your biceps. The same is true for your triceps. No wonder your arms all sore and small. They are so over trained. Follow the principles contained in this course and in time your arms will get Brutally Huge and look like legs!

18 INCH FOREARMS

Thank you for buying this course. This course will show you how to get forearms that are so huge that people will be afraid to shake your hand when you stick it out near them. Your forearms will look like bowling pins, and oversize drumsticks. Large massive forearms are essential for the complete look to your arms. Nothing looks more ridiculous than someone who has huge upper arms, and has tiny little forearms. Large forearms are intimidating. My forearms extended are 16.25", and in the gooseneck position my forearms are about 17".

Massive forearms are an awesome sight indeed! Functionally massive and powerful forearms are a must if you are to work your back, biceps, rows, deadlifts, and other exercises properly, where a strong grip is needed. How many times have you had to terminate a set of deadlifts, or 400 lb shrugs because the bar was slipping out of your fingers? How many times have bicep curls been terminated short of failure because your forearms were going numb, and your grip was giving out? This shouldn't happen and when it does it is only ruining the set for the particular body part you are training. Something must be done, and intelligent forearm training will solve your problems bars slipping from your grip, and spindly looking forearms. Furthermore, don't be surprised if when you start working forearms on a regular basis your upper arms pop on a quick 1\4 to a 1\2". I have this theory about growth. One of the things that of course make you grow, is training to failure. Something else that makes you grow is engorging a muscle with as much blood as possible. So when you work biceps first and pump all that blood into them, they are maybe a 1\2" bigger during the workout; however half of your arm is still empty. When you train forearms after biceps even more blood must go through the biceps to get into the forearms. So now you have a lot more blood in the biceps, and indeed the whole arm. Also have you ever noticed that when you work forearms after biceps and go home that your whole arm stays pumped longer than if you didn't work the forearms? So I believe that forearm work has an indirect effect on a lot of muscles that you train, not just themselves, the forearms. For example, you are bent over doing 300lb rows for your lats and when the reps for lats get tougher you start cheating to grind out those last impossible reps, and you can't because the bar is rolling out of your fingers, and you have to concentrate more on your failing grip than the lats you are supposed to be working. That just limits your lat potential!

There are three kinds of muscles in the forearms:

1) the muscles responsible for Flexion of the wrist
2) the muscles responsible for extension of the wrists
3) the muscles responsible for gripping

If you clench your fist and bend your hand back and forth you will see certain muscles and tendons moving in your forearms. If however you put your forearm out straight with your palm facing the ceiling, and close your fingers tight and relax them back and forth you will see other things moving in there. Also if you look at the outside of your forearm in the mirror as you close and open your fist you will see cords of muscle moving around in sequence. This should show you that there are the gripping muscles and the wrist flexion muscles. A lot of people treat forearm training like it is a real inconvenience, but they are the ones who have small forearms. Then there are the people who feel guilty about not doing forearms, and so they grab a 30lb chrome fixed barbell and do a few sloppy sets, so they can say they worked them. Forearms are capable of getting very strong and large if they are trained hard and properly. In this course I am going to show you the techniques that have worked for me, and that will give similar improvements for you too.

If you were hanging on the edge of a cliff for dear life; how long do you think you could hang there if you had to, and there was molten lava below you? A study that I did at college with a bunch of friends showed that most people can hang about 45 seconds to 2 minutes depending on who they were, how heavy they were, and other variables. I will make a bet with you. I'll bet that you can't hang on to a bar for 5 minutes, and I don't care if you hang one hand at a time or both hands together, or underhand, overhand, or taking turns with hands while you are hanging there in mid air. The rule is simple hang there anyway you can without your feet touching the floor or helping you in any way. As you can see grip strength is very important if you ever had to use it.

One of the best ways I know to build grip strength, is after your biceps exercises, do 2 sets of hanging from a chinning bar. On the first set use your bodyweight and just hang there for 30 seconds. The only rule you have to follow is: squeeze the bar much, much harder than you have to in order to hang there. Don't pace yourself and squeeze that bar as hard as you can. Your fingers should be turning white. When you get down you shouldn't be able to open your fingers easily if you did the set right. On the second set hang as much weight as you can around your waist and hang for 30 seconds, if possible. When you can do that add more weight next workout. Don't be afraid and start off with a puny 40 lb dumbbell. Don't play around with them or they won't grow. When you are hanging there imagine that your life depends on it. That will help you finish the set.

One of the other purposes of this course was to show you the many different exercises you can do for your forearms. Most people think that all there is are wrist curls, and maybe dumbbell wrist curls. There are so many other exercises than the two I have just mentioned. I could think of a dozen or more exercises that I could tell you and I will. There are lots of principles that you need to utilize if you want to get huge forearms.

1) You should only work your forearms when you work your biceps, and if you are advanced, that may be once every 4th or 5th day.

2) When you are a beginner you should do only 3 sets of one particular exercise, nothing changes if you are intermediate or advanced,

except you may find 2 sets each for the flexor and extensors is enough (i.e.- reverse wrist curls and wrist curls).

3) Make sure that you are also doing heavy exercises for the rest of your body as this will have an indirect effect on the gripping muscles.

4) Train them as hard and as heavy as any other muscle, don't act like they are a nuisance.

5) Increase the weight whenever possible

6) Forearms love high reps which induce lots of pain. The more pain you can generate and tolerate, the more they will grow.

7) Cramping, flexing, and tensing in different positions during, before, and after sets will promote vascularity and increase the pump.

8) When you are doing forearms and you have reached the point where full reps are no longer possible; then continue on with partials until you can no longer even twitch the bar, and then try to hold on to it, and squeeze it as hard as possible.

9) Whenever you get sick of one exercise or it no longer produces any results then switch to another one.

Now I will detail my favorite forearm exercises.

Reverse Barbell Curls-This exercise affects the Brachioradialis, which is the large upper outer portion of the forearm. Grab a bar with a 10-14" wide grip. With your palms facing forward, and your elbows at your sides; raise the bar upward, cramp the muscle, and then slowly lower it. If a straight bar hurts your wrists, use a kamber curl bar instead. Honestly, I feel you won't even need to directly work this muscle due to all the indirect stimulation from rows, etc. But if you do, limit it to 1-2 sets.

Reverse Wrist Curls-This exercise affects the Extensor Carpi Ulnaris, and the Extensor Digitorum. Sitting on a bench with your forearms resting on your thighs, and your palms facing upwards; let the weight down and raise it up as far as you can and feel it cramp up on you. One or two pumping sets to failure is sufficient.

Standing Reverse Wrist Curls- This is a peak contraction movement. Start with the weight hanging at arms length, in front of your thighs. Your palms will be facing your thighs. The key here is to raise the weight up thru the short range of movement as high as you can and hold the count for 2 seconds on each rep. This exercise works the Extensor Carpi Radialis

Longus, and the Extensor Digitorium. Once again, 2 sets is sufficient.

Standing Barbell Wrist Curls- This movement is done with a thumbless grip, bar in front of the thighs, palms facing forward, and the arms hanging down straight. It is a short range of movement exercise, an awkward movement that hits the Flexor Carpi Radialis. High reps and tension are the keys here. Cramp it up at the top as hard as you can, hold for 3 seconds, and slowly lower. Do no more than 2 sets here.

Standing wrist curls with barbell behind the waist. Grab a bar off a rack, and let it hang behind your hamstrings with your palms facing away from your body. Cramp the weight up as high as it'll go and hold for 2 to 3 seconds before lowering. Do high reps to failure. This exercise will work the grip, and hit the Palmaris Longus, Flexor Carpi Ulnaris, And the Flexor Digitorium Profundus. You can get very strong on this movement so don't be afraid to use heavy weights. I have gone up to 295 for 6 reps.

Hanging with additional weight- I've already mentioned this one. It stimulates every muscle in the forearms Use as much weight as possible for 2 sets maximum.

Dumbbell Wrist Curl- with the forearm resting on your thighs, and the palms facing up; curl the weight for the fullest reps possible and do partials when full ones are no longer possible. This exercise works the Flexor Carpi Radialis. Two sets are more than enough.

Dumbbell Reverse Wrist Curls- This is the reverse of the above movement and it hits the Extensor Carpi Radialis Longus. Two sets is all you need.

Standing Wrist Curls with the hands in front of the waist and the palms facing your thighs. This exercise affects the Flexor Carpi Ulnaris. Do 2 sets, high reps to failure, and go as heavy as possible.

Reminder, do not perform all the above exercise, but only pick one for wrist curls, and one for the reverse wrist curl movement. If you choose hanging from a bar as your forearm exercise, then do not do any regular wrist curls as you will overtrain the area and not grow. Follow the principles in this section, and your forearms will indeed be Brutally thick!

BRUTAL ABDOMINALS

Many people think that there is some mysterious process to building abs. In my opinion there is only two parts to getting outrageous looking abs: 1) building the muscle thickness, and 2) dieting off the existing fat, so that the abs can show clearly. Abs grow so easy there is no excuse not to have them. All it takes is intelligence, desire, and proper training. Abs only contract in one direction. Abs are not complicated like the Deltoids. In this course, I will outline the routines, exercises, sets, reps, and theories that you will use to blast your abs. First let us cover some of misconceptions concerning abdominal work. I think that one of the biggest myths is that working your abs hard will cause you to over train the rest of your body. Indeed, I've heard that doing a 1000 resp can have a negative effect on the rest of your body. However, we won't do that here. Psychologically speaking, if your waist were tight and small; your upper body would feel huge. Another myth is that abs need hundreds or thousands of reps to develop. Some people, unfortunately, train this way every day. Abs are a muscle just like the thighs, or arms. Therefore, you should train them the same way. You wouldn't do a 100 reps per set on your lats, so don't train your abs that way either. When training abs you are not trying to set endurance records. When you train your abs train them to failure using the heaviest weight possible. Whenever you can do the required number of reps, add more weight the next workout. You'll never get abs with inch deep ridges in them doing sets of a 100 reps; only heavy resistance will do that. All those reps will only flatten out and over train your abs. The best principles that you can use to build your abs are:

1) Overload Principle
2) Low Sets
3) Train to failure
4) Supersets or trisets
5) Peak contraction on all reps

Another myth is that of spot reduction. Some people think that doing thousands of sit-ups will burn fat off their midriffs. This is false and untrue. Fat is burned evenly over the whole body. If you are losing fat off your gut; then you are also losing fat off your other body parts too. If you have an inch of fat on your arms, but you also have 4 inches of fat on your waist; it stands to reason that your arms will get ripped before your abs do. Also, don't waste your time doing lots of stupid broomstick twists thinking that you will burn off your "love handles". However, lowering your fats, and calories combined with aerobics will melt off fat real fast. In the next few pages you will find many routines to blast your abs. Your number one enemy is overtraining. Don't ever do more exercises, than is listed. Remember your abs get a lot of indirect effect from other exercises like tricep press downs. Remember it's exercise that stimulates the abs to grow, while rest allows growth to happen, and diet allows them to show.

Actual routines

Beginners - Only work your abs twice a week. Do only one exercise for the abs, and perform only three sets of that exercise. Perform a warm up set, a medium set, and an all out gut busting set. Of course, you will be adding weight each set. Furthermore, try to add weight each and every workout, or whenever possible. This kind of training will lay down a good foundation of strength, and thicken up the actual rows of rectus abdominis muscle. If you don't have any you will soon. Here are some sample routines:

Routines:
A) Decline Weighted Crunches   3 sets of 10, 8, and 6 reps
B) Weighted Leg Raises   3 sets of 15, 12, and 10 reps
C) Weighted Situps   3

sets of 10,8, and 6 reps
D) Roman Chair Situps — 3 sets of 10,8, and 6 reps
E) Kneeling Rope Pulldowns — 3 sets of 12,8, and 6 reps
F) Hanging Leg Raises — 3 sets of 15,10, and6 reps
G) Incline Leg Raises — 3 sets of 10,8, and 6 reps
H) Weighted Crunches With Inversion Boots 3 sets 10,8,6 reps

All these routines aren't just listed as course filler so I could advertise 40 or 50 gut wrenching routines, no, they were all listed to make you think, and to make you realize that there is more to ab development than just doing sit-ups for the rest of your life.

Most people will never develop thick rows of abs doing 1000's of repetitions. Remember, you are trying to build muscle thickness not set endurance records. Always do low sets, low reps, and with heavy weights, and fierce determination. As you do your exercises such as crunches; don't just sit up with your torso as straight as a board; instead put your chin to your chest, and curl your torso inward and forward at the same time. Imagine yourself as being one of those rolly-bugs that turns into a ball. Furthermore, doing stiff sit-ups has hurt more than one person's lower back. Injury results when a large internal muscle pulls on your spine when you do a stiff sit-up. This muscle is called the Psoas Major. The surface muscles or the rectus abdominis comes into play when you curl your torso inward. Always do slow movements and maintain tension on the abs. Try to achieve and feel a deep pain. Also, at the finish of each rep, crunch the abs as hard as possible; this will help put peaks on the rows of muscle. Never just flop over at the finish of a rep; all you are doing then is resting. You can rest after the set. During the set you must be in pain, and the more you delve into that pain and love it, the more you will grow.

Intermediates

At this level of development you can do two exercises for the abs. You may continue working the abs twice a week, and do two exercises for two sets each. As with the beginner routines you will still add weight whenever possible.

<u>Sample routines</u>
A) Incline Leg Raises-2 sets of 15, 10 reps
   Weighted Crunches-2 sets of 8, 6 reps

B) Leg Raises 2 sets of-12, and 8 reps
   Decline Crunches-2 sets of 6, and 6 reps

C) Alternate Leg Raises-2 sets of 20, and 15 reps
   Roman Chair Crunches-2 sets of 10, and 8 reps

D) Rope Pull downs-2 sets of 15, and 10 reps
   Weighted Sit-ups-2 sets of 6, and 6 reps

E) Weighted Db sidebends-2 sets of 15, and 10 reps
   Hanging Weighted Sit-ups-2 sets of 8, and 6 reps

F) Weighted Roman Chair Twists-2 sets of 10, and 6 rep
   Hanging Leg Raises-2 sets of 8, and 6 reps

G) Hanging Knee-ins-2 sets of 20, and 15 reps
   Steep Incline Sit-ups-2 sets of 8, and 6 reps

There is no limit to the different combinations of exercises you can do. If you had the 6 best exercises that would give you 6 x 5 x 4 x 3 x 2 x 1 = 720 different routines; this meaning that you should never get bored.

Advanced

At the advanced level you will still need to do only two or three exercises that will work different areas of the abs. At the advanced levels you will also want to start shaping the abs, as well as paying attention to the intercostals. The intercostals are the muscles between the ribs. The Serratus will also have to be developed, but I really consider them to be part of Lat training and can be hit with the dumbbell pullovers. At the advanced levels developing your intercostals will give you that complete, polished, and professional look. Also at the advanced stages you still want to increase the poundage whenever possible, but you will want to pay more attention to form. You must go for that afterburner pain, and crunch the abs as hard as possible. You will also need to start doing supersets and trisets. This will serve three purposes: 1) to save time and 2) to raise the intensity levels and 3) to promote a pump that you will never feel from doing straight sets.

Furthermore, at this stage your abs are probably too strong and stubborn to respond to the monotony of straight sets anyway. Listed first are some example triset routines, and the muscles they affect.

Routine A
Leg Raises -2 sets 10,10reps lower abs
Weighted Crunches-2 sets 8, 6 reps upper abs
Angled Crunches-2 sets 6, 6 reps intercostals

Routine B
Incline Leg Raises-2 sets 10,8 reps lower abs
Decline Crunches-2 sets 8,8 reps upper abs
Angled Leg Raises-2 sets 6,6 reps intercostals, obliques

Routine C
Hanging Leg Raise -2 sets 10 reps lower abs, hip flexors
Weighted Sit-ups-2 sets 8,6 reps upper abs
Decline Angled Crunch-2 sets 6,6 reps upper intercostals

Routine D
Twists-2 sets of 10 reps obliques, intercostals
Roman Crunches-2 sets 8,8reps upper abs
Hanging Angled Knee ups-2 sets 6,6 reps lower abs, intercostals

The above listed routines are done in straight set fashion. When you are performing supersets, pick only two exercises that affect different areas of the abs, and do them both in a row, in a nonstop fashion. Perform only 2 supersets as the pump and ache that you will experience is unlike anything you've ever felt.

Furthermore there is always that chance of overtraining; actually it is more than a chance it will happen, and you know what happens when you over train: no growth, and possible injuries. Trisets are an advanced technique that will not only thicken your abs, but will flush, pump, striate, and sharpen every muscle in the area. A triset is performed by doing 3 different exercises, for only one set each. Do all three nonstop. This series will constitute 1 triset. Do only 2 trisets as they are so intense that performing any more will result in severe soreness, overtraining, and possible injury.

Next up the ladder of abdominal stimulation are quadsets, and giant sets. Now, I am not the inventor of these techniques (i.e. giant, super, tri-, or quadsets); I am just putting them into a system that I feel I developed called the Brutally Huge system, which is based on under training and the inability of the body to ingest and respond from large amounts of exercise, or what I'd call gross overtraining. In a quadset, you do 4 exercises in a row nonstop until you've completed one quadset series. Giant sets are 5 exercises in a row. Giant sets and Quadsets are really pre-contest regimens for cutting up, and shaping the abs. They shouldn't be done for more than 4 weeks as they will fry your nerves. High intensity doesn't just over train the muscles; it also really puts a drain on the systems, and subsystems that recuperate the muscles; such as your endocrine and nervous system. High intensity methods prolonged for long periods of time can really stress your adrenal cortex, which can rapidly lead to overtraining. Below is an example quadset:

Twists-1 set 10 reps Obliques
Weighted leg raises-1 sets 6 reps-lower abs
Weighted crunches-1 set 6 reps-upper abs
Angled Crunches-1 set 6 reps-intercostals

The above constitutes 1 quadset. Perform this sequence only twice. Giant sets are 5 exercises done in a row. Below is a typical giant set:

Hanging Leg Raises-1 set 10 reps-lower abs
Twists-1 set 8 reps-obliques
Angled Crunches-1 set 6 reps-intercostals
Weighted sit-ups-1 set 6 reps-middle abs
Decline crunches -1 set 4 reps -upper abs

Try the above techniques for your next contest. You won't believe the results.

Warning: You should not perform this or any intense routine without a physician's checkup first.

Record of Measurements

Date	Thighs	Waist	Chest	Biceps	Calves	Weight

NOTES